BETTER AT THE BROKEN PLACES

By
Jeffrey R. Pickering

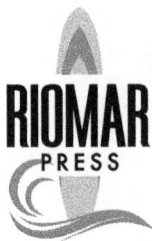

RIOMAR
PRESS

For Stephanie, Colin, Grant, and Olivia.
Always.

Acknowledgements

This book began more than 30 years ago with a 16-year-old boy crouched behind home plate, fastball inside corner – a crack of the bat, a violent play at the plate, and a world that would change forever. In the pages that follow, I tell a difficult story that would likely not have been written if it were not for . . .

. . . the private, professional medical and behavioral health care provided by my primary care physician, my therapists, and the staff of The Green Shoe Foundation. Thank you for answering my call for help and for restoring my trust in medicine.

. . . the rock-solid support of the first few friends I talked to about my experience of childhood sexual abuse, especially Tung, Ingrid, Kari, Tom, Tania, Gray, Adam, Hope, Albert, Herb, and Harry. Thank you for being there when I needed it most.

. . . the hundreds of people who read along with the daily posts I published on a serial blog beginning in February 2020, in an effort to continue healing, to help others, and to pursue justice. I was able to achieve each of these because of you.

. . . the wise legal counsel I received from Michael, Joe, Matt, and Michael.

. . . the respectful, dignified, empowering opportunity that a series of public radio interviews provided. Thank you, Richard, and Rogers.

. . . the creative guidance of my writing coach, Cole, the superior editing by Jennifer and Susan, and the design and production wizardry of Glenn.

. . . the generous TEDx audience. Terrifying but well worth the experience.

. . . the occasional cold one with a brother.

. . . the ocean and the waves.

. . . the unconditional love of Stephanie, Colin, Olivia, Grant . . . and Tilly (woof).

. . . the brave men and women who have reached out to say "me too." I believe you. I am so sorry that it happened to you. I am here for you.

Table of Contents

Monday, October 16, 2017

The online surf report for my local break at the pier in Vero Beach, Florida, did not give me much hope for an after-work surf session by the time I was wrapping up my day at the office. "Three foot and choppy" was all I had to look forward to.

Like most days, I had already checked the surf report multiple times since waking up using Surfline, a mobile app that provides detailed information about wave height, wind, tides, water temperature, swell direction, and future forecasts. "Know before you go" is the company's reliable mantra, and on nearly every occasion the information was right on.

Without much to look forward to, my mind drifted. I searched other favorite destinations from past surf trips taken around the world:

Kawaihae Harbor on Hawaii Island's northwest coast, "fair"; Salt Creek in Dana Point, California, "firing"; Pavones on Costa Rica's Pacific coast near the Panamanian border, "swell building"; Lahinch Beach on Ireland's west coast in County Cork, "massive, steely-gray and cold."

When I got home, I stepped out on to the balcony to check the waves with my own eyes. It was an age-old ritual practiced for generations by surfers around the globe: a hopeful, reverent genuflection I first learned as a young boy, forever connecting me to my tribe and a cosmic push and pull that created the waves. I closed my eyes, drew a deep breath of salt air, and let my mind drift toward the sea and a decades-old memory of the first time I tried surfing.

As a Florida native, time at the ocean had always been part of my life. Surfing, however, began for me in 1983, the summer I turned 10 years old while on family vacation a few hours up the coast in the tiny hamlet of New Smyrna Beach. It was a June afternoon when I screwed up the courage and made the decision to leave the inflatable canvas raft behind to try surfing for the first time in my life.

This first surf session was a moment that had possessed me since the summer of 1981, the first time I walked into the new surf shop in the strip mall around the corner from my older cousin Matt's house in Casselberry, Florida. Despite being an hour's drive away from the ocean and wedged between a dry cleaners and a furniture store, Belitz Surf Company felt as if the beach and all the trappings of surf culture had just landed in my backyard.

The intoxicating scent of coconut oil and Sex Wax blended with the punk rock sounds of Agent Orange and TSOL. A familiar latch-key-kid language coming from the frenetic scene of sun-kissed look-alikes clad in Sundek surf trunks and slip-on Vans, huddled around a massive television where a grainy VHS tape played footage of legendary surfers Shaun Thompson and Mark Richards dropping into a tandem tube ride at Off-the-Wall on Oahu's North Shore.

This sweet euphoria propelled me as I walked down to the beach rental truck from our condo at Moontide and handed over a five-dollar bill to pay for an hour's rental of a real fiberglass surfboard. It was a blue twin-fin with several years-worth of gray, pasty wax built up on the deck. The rails were thick, with several patches where dings had been repaired. The leash was a simple nylon cord with a loop at the end to attach to my left foot.

I walked to the water's edge, posing with the board tucked under my right arm exactly how I had observed in the pages of Surfer magazine. It might have been enough just to stand there, catching the eye of a passerby and flashing a look that told them I was different than anyone they had ever laid eyes on, I knew better. That's what poseurs and kooks do – not me. I laid down on the board, paddled out and in the sixty minutes of frothing that followed, I became a surfer.

Thirty-six years later, as I stood at the railing of my balcony and looked east, I was surprised to see a swell building on the outer reef despite the conditions reported by Surfline. My wife, Stephanie, had an eye on the kids, three-bean chili was in the crockpot, cornbread was in the oven, and the ocean's surface looked like corduroy on the horizon. The sun had already set, but there was still enough light left to get in a ride or two before dinner.

The air and ocean water temperatures were the same at 72 degrees. I threw on my favorite pair of Patagonia boardshorts and a long-sleeved Yulex wetsuit top to keep the chill off. With an hour or so left before high tide, I quickly rubbed wax on my 9-foot Fletcher Chouinard Designs HP longboard. The extra length helped get through the deep, swampy section between the outside and inside reefs.

I entered the water on the north side of the pier and paddled out. Barnacles clung to the concrete pilons. A few baitfish broke the surface. I caught three lefts, riding the last one into the shadow of the pier and onto the beach, a stolen bit of solitude and serenity at the start of a busy week.

Showered and fed, I settled onto the couch with my wife, Stephanie, to watch a recording of NBC Nightly News with Lester Holt. Our 13-year-old son, Colin, cleared the table, and our 12-year-old daughter, Olivia, loaded the dishwasher. Our 4-year-old son, Grant, played quietly on the floor with Legos and Magnatiles. It was a nightly ritual, a dose of comfort in an otherwise full life of a busy family of five.

The evening's headlines included reports of a joint press conference President Donald Trump held with Senate Majority Leader Mitch McConnell, a guilty plea from Army Sergeant Bowe Bergdahl for desertion of his platoon while serving in Afghanistan, California wildfires, and a final story on some new troubles for movie mogul Harvey Weinstein.

This last story about Weinstein horrified us. It was being reported as a new rallying cry was catching fire on social media. Many women had begun posting "#metoo" if they had ever faced sexual assault or harassment from anyone. So many men in power were being accused of disgusting acts of sexual misconduct, some of which had gone unreported for years. Others had been simply dismissed, tethering victims to an invisible fuse ignited by these new accusations against Weinstein.

With little ears around, we moved into our bedroom and took a deeper dive online, pouring over story after depraved story of sexual assault and molestation. One set of news reports was particularly horrifying – a July 11th guilty plea to child pornography charges by a 54-year-old Michigan doctor named Larry Nasser who was also facing more than 100 claims of sexual assault by women and girls that dated back as far as 1998. Most were gymnasts, and several were current and former Olympians.

Sitting on our bed, leaning back on pillows against the padded headboard with the sound of waves crashing against the pier outside our bedroom window, I asked Stephanie if she had ever experienced anything similar. She replied with a flat out, "No." Yes, she had encountered many guys who were jerks, either in the workplace or a social setting, but she had never been sexually assaulted.

I was getting tired, and this is where I thought we would leave the conversation for the night until Stephanie asked, "What about you?"

The question startled me. It prompted an involuntary reflex to repel the mere idea that something like that had ever happened to me. I sensed the words "of course not" on the tip of my tongue.

Then, out of nowhere, the room spun with the same vertigo flood that comes with a two-wave hold down in the ocean: a tumbling revolution of dark, light, dark, light with a mechanical cadence that reminded me of an old-school filmstrip reel I used as a child at the Winter Park Public Library.

A familiar doctor's face framed by a bowtie.

Slow turn of a black screen.

3

A red and white ointment tube.
Slow turn of a black screen.
An examination table.
Slow turn of a black screen.
An ungloved hand.
Slow turn of a black screen.
A bright, thin green stripe on the waistband of a boy's underwear.
Slow turn of a black screen.
A blinding white light.

I was gagging on my last breath before a seafoam inhalation, inches below the surface. I did not know why I was seeing and remembering these images, but it terrified me. The concerned look on Stephanie's face told me so.

Safe on her shore, suddenly, the memories began to come together. The familiar doctor's face framed by glasses and a bowtie was *my* child-hood doctor. The red and white ointment tube was one of the supplies that was arranged on the counter next to the examination table that *I* laid on. The ungloved hand was *my* doctor's ungloved hand, attached to the fingers where the ointment was applied. The thin green stripe was on the waistband of *my* underwear. The blinding white light was being shined from the corner of a pitch-black room in *my* eyes, by *my* doctor. I broke down in tears and told her everything I was remembering, the images that were surfacing that had been submerged deep in my psyche for 30 years.

I told Stephanie that I remembered being treated for a knee injury by an Orlando, Florida, pediatric orthopedic surgeon when I was sixteen years old during my junior year in high school. I told her that I remembered an accident in a baseball game; red clay in my hair; a hospital visit from my high school girlfriend, Ana, and her sister; a knee surgery; an uncomfortable cast, crutches, knee braces and months of recovery. I told her that I remembered the doctor putting his ungloved finger in my rectum on multiple occasions. I told her that I remembered the doctor fondling my genitals. I told her that I remembered being photographed in the nude without a parent present. I remembered all of this being done under the guise of medical care.

Now I was 44 years old, married, a proud father of three beautiful children, living on the ocean, surfing every day, at the peak of my career, and for the first time in my life, I had just told someone that I remembered being sexually abused as a child . . . by my doctor.

Stephanie and I spent a few minutes searching the internet for information about this doctor, William P. Zink, M.D. One of the first search results that appeared indicated that he was affiliated with the athletics department at Orlando's Edgewater High School, the public high school

4

that was my father's alma mater and located less than a mile from the private Catholic high school that I graduated from.

We also found a poorly designed website with his name and a header that read "Orlando Pediatric Sports Medicine." The website included information about his office staff and hours of operation, along with a quote below his headshot photo that read:

"Recognized as one of the most highly respected pediatric orthopedic practitioners in Central Florida for the treatment of youth sports injuries. Each year we see hundreds of patients ranging in age from infancy through young adult. These patients seek specialized medical and surgical care for a variety of musculoskeletal diseases and injuries."

Finally, from the listing on the corporate website, it looked as if Dr. Zink was on the medical staff of AdventHealth with privileges to perform surgery at its main hospital in Orlando. This is the same hospital system where my father is employed. It is also the same hospital where my two older children were born.

I could not believe it, thinking that Dr. Zink must have been at least 70 years old. He should have been retired by now, but he wasn't.

I could not believe it, thinking about more of what I remembered him doing to me just days before I left for college He should have been in prison, but he wasn't.

He ... was ... still ... practicing.

1
Trust

I grew up in Winter Park, Florida, a winter retreat founded in the late 1800's by wealthy northerners seeking refuge from harsh winters and a tranquil place to rest and relax. The city is famous for its stately oak trees, brick-lined streets, and historic homes of people like architect Gamble Rogers and sculptor Albin Polacek. Among the city's charms is the 999-acre Winter Park Chain of Lakes; Florida's oldest college, Rollins College; the Morse Museum housing the world's most comprehensive collection of works by Louis Comfort Tiffany; its own Central Park; and the boutique hotel The Alfond Inn, a luxury mashup of art, farm-to-table dining, and bespoke accommodations that has become the new town hall.

I am the oldest of three sons, raised by middle class parents; my mom, a retired critical care nurse, and my father, retired from the auto-motive repair industry and now in his second career as a nuclear medicine technologist. My parents are good, hard-working people whose livelihoods and ability to provide for our family were built on trust.

Beyond family life and school, two institutions dominated my child-hood: the Catholic church and baseball. Both contributed significantly to the man I have become.

As an active member of St. Margaret Mary Catholic Church, I served as altar boy, youth group leader, work-camp participant, and homeless shelter volunteer. For several summers during and after high school, I traveled on mission trips to rural Appalachia and to the Dominican Republic to work and to build relationships among the poor, marginalized residents of those places. These were the activities that shaped my sense of service and fostered my belief in a higher power.

The nuns I knew were kind, albeit hard-nosed, advocates for causes on behalf of the poor and marginalized. Sister Ann, Sister Gail, and Sister Theresa led our diocesan office of farmworker ministry and taught me how to work for social justice.

The priests I knew were like God. My pastor, Father Richard Walsh, and my high school chaplain, Father Leo Hodges, were good men who were strong role models for me. I trusted their wisdom and followed their examples of Christian love.

As an athlete, my first love was baseball. Catcher was the only position I ever played, and the baseball diamonds of Winter Park Little League are where I learned how to win, how to lose, and most importantly, how to lead.

My childhood T-ball team was sponsored by Golden Corral Steakhouse. I wore a bright orange jersey and white sliding pants. My first glove was a tan leather Rawlings fielder's mitt that fit just right. Our team's equipment was carried in an Army green canvas duffel bag. Inside were bats, balls, batting helmets, and a poor-fitting set of catcher's equipment that included shin guards made of plastic and worn leather, a quilted cloth chest protector, and a facemask that smelled like shoe polish. I was in heaven.

After T-ball, my minor league team was sponsored by Middleton Pest Control, a local company owned by our coach. Green jersey, same white sliding pants. I was nine years old and needed a bigger glove. It was a black leather Mizuno fielder's mitt. The catcher's mitt I used during practices and games was provided by the league and shared with the team, along with the other contents of the equipment bag.

Our "secret weapon" on the Middleton Pest Control team was a six-foot tall, left-handed tomboy named Shannon Carrell Gridley who played first base. She was the only member of the team who hit any homeruns that season. The coach's son, Jason, had the best arm, but he could get wild on occasion throwing sidearm pitches in the dirt. He hit a fair share of batters, too, which usually resulted in a crying fit in the dugout by the time he got out of the inning. This was also the year that another pitcher, Shane Moncrief, took a come-back line drive to his forehead. The doctors said it was a standard concussion, but I do not believe he ever fully recovered.

When I turned ten years old, I moved up to the major leagues. We were the Angels, and Joe Russell was my coach. Coach Russell was drafted as a pitcher by the Texas Rangers in the third round of the 1974 Major League Baseball draft. He was the first person to really "teach" me the game of baseball. He treated each of us boys almost as if we were adults, with respect and as if we had one job to do: hustle. The wins would follow. These lessons stayed with me as I matured through the ranks of recreational Little League to the competitive world of varsity sports and beyond.

The two years I spent playing on Joe Russell's team was the first time in my life that I can remember feeling the experience of growing up, like I was more than just a kid. The major leagues were also the first time that players were allowed to steal bases. No leading off, but once the pitch crossed home plate, base runners were allowed to make an attempt. This challenged me as a catcher.

When I first entered the league at ten years old, my throwing arm was not very strong. I had difficulty making an accurate throw to second base, sometimes bouncing the ball before the bag and other times sending it into center field. By the end of my second season in the major leagues, however, my arm was stronger. Fewer stolen bases were recorded against our Angels team. I made the All-Star Team that year, and in our last regular season game, which was a replay of a previous rain-out, I hit the only home run of my entire baseball career. A two-run dinger off a hanging curveball hurled by freckle-faced Taylor Hart.

The next year, my Little League season coincided with my first year at Glenridge Junior High School. I got cut trying out for the school team and was drafted by the Pony League White Sox. This was the first level that teams played on a regulation-size baseball field. The pitcher's mound was farther away from home plate, the bases were 90 feet apart, and runners were allowed to lead off. It was the first time where base-running really came into play, and it was everything our coach obsessed about.

Our White Sox coach was the most unlikely person to inspire confidence in a group of thirteen-year-old boys. On practice days, he would arrive at the field in a white Dodge Duster and shout at one of us to meet him at his car to carry the equipment. Rock, paper, scissors, and whoever lost would spend the next ten minutes turning a foot-long flathead screwdriver in the lock of the Duster's trunk while the coach placed both hands on the trunk and pressed down with all of his 135 pounds until the trunk popped open.

Equipment delivered, practice would begin the same way every day: meet at first base and practice leading off – shoulder-width sidestep, shoulder-width sidestep, another if you could. Hands open, fingers wiggling, arms dangling toward the ground, a shout of "back" by the coach, and the runner would need to dive back to the bag and reach for the back left corner, hopefully avoiding the first-baseman's swipe.

After every team member tried, we would turn our attention to an exercise our coach called "rounding the bag." Start with a lead off from first base, we would take off running toward second base, and as you approached second base round the bag in an arc that would put us on a direct course to reach third base by running the shortest possible distance.

Unfortunately, the offensive performance of our White Sox team that year was unproductive. All those baserunning skills were never put to much use, as we struggled all season long to get on base. It was the last year I remember certain kids playing Little League. Some changed to a different sport or found other interests like the school orchestra or the local theatre. Other kids started drinking alcohol or got into drugs, sometimes doing so in the same wooded preserve that bordered our Little League fields within earshot of the dugout and concession stand chatter. One boy died in a freak bicycle accident, resulting in a memorial sportsmanship award that I received the following year.

Eighth grade at Glenridge Junior High School was magical. The year began with my first season on the football team, my first girlfriend Becky, and my first experience of making the cut for the Lions baseball team in the spring. Jimmy Argeros was the ninth grader starting as catcher, with a cannon for an arm and a productive bat, which meant slim chances that I would see much playing time. It didn't matter to me. Instead of being one of "them," now I was one of "us."

Our coach, Sid Hair, was a no-nonsense operator whose mere presence on the field and generally sour disposition commanded respect from all of us. His adult son Todd was the wild-eyed assistant coach who ran our practices and enforced Coach Hair's redneck discipline both on and off the field. It was all "yes sir" and "no sir." Back talk was a cardinal sin. A lesson one teammate, Billy, learned the hard way from the wrong end of an open-handed slap to his face that ended practice early, along with Todd's coaching career, after a visit from the Winter Park police.

Coach Hair's youngest son, Clay, was our ace pitcher and resident team playboy. Herbert "Butch" Lilly was our first baseman and homerun leader. Keith Gill, the team's sole Black player, was a picture of strength and grace in our last game of the season, pitching a complete game in my one start behind the plate as catcher as the other half of the battery. We won, delivering a fitting defeat on the home field of Robert E. Lee Junior High School.

During both my freshman and sophomore years of high school, I tried out but did not make the varsity teams. I was disappointed to not be playing catcher for the Winter Park Wildcats but stayed active by playing for the Blue Jays in my final two seasons of Little League. Rick "Spanky" Snyder coached my team to a league championship and an All-Star Team that beat Maitland's standout players Russ McBryde, Robby Robinson, and their crew of cross-town rivals in our final game. We were boys who had become men: winners who were ready to take on the world.

It was the summer that I turned sixteen years old. It was also the time when I made my decision to leave Winter Park High School and transfer to the private Bishop Moore Catholic High School for my junior and senior years. Bishop Moore was my mother's alma mater and a few blocks away from the public high school my father attended. It felt familiar to me. It was a smaller school, attended by a few friends from church, and came with a chance to be the starting catcher for the Hornets. It was the first "adult" decision I ever made, and one that has paid tremendous dividends ever since through lifelong friendships and a sense of finally belonging.

Despite how proud I was for this conscious choice of a better path for my future, at the time I would have had no way of knowing that this very mature decision also put me on a collision course with a horror that no child is equipped to face. A terror that I might have seen coming if it were foreshadowed by the kind of ominous thriller-movie soundtrack that most teenaged boys knew by heart.

John Williams composed the double bass F-F sharp alert that told me that Jaws' prehistoric maw was just below the surface. When I heard it, I got out of the water. Harry Manfredini recorded the staccato "ki, ki, ki, ma, ma, ma" to accompany Jason's Friday the 13th stride. When I heard it, I locked the door.

My newfound confidence, however, was about to be destroyed by the worst kind of monster. One that does not look or sound or smell like a monster at all. One that strikes without warning:

One with a degree from the Louisiana State University of Medicine; one with a license to practice medicine in my home state of Florida; one with a certification from the American Board of Orthopedic Surgery; one with a membership in the Orange County Medical Society; one with a wife and children of his own and a pleasant, eager-to-please demeanor; one who has taken an oath to "do no harm" and to preserve the finest traditions of a calling that, if practiced with fidelity, all but guarantees a reward to experience the joy of healing those who seek his help.

When I heard this, I did not run. I did not hide. I did not scream or cry for help. When I heard all of this, instead, I became his patient.

2
Broken

arrived at school on the morning of Tuesday, February 13, 1990, feeling excited. Our first home game was scheduled for that afternoon against the Mt. Dora High School Hurricanes, and the lineup card would be posted on the coach's classroom door for the team to check before the first bell rang. After a disappointing football season the previous fall, those of us who were two-sport athletes were eager to redeem ourselves.

Seniors Beau Delaporte and Peter Egan were already outside coach's classroom door inspecting the white three-by-five card taped to the inside of the square glass window. "Pickering, catcher, batting seventh," Delaporte shouted. "You're going to have to be a dog back there, Pick," Egan said. "PK is on the mound."

"PK" stood for knuckleballer Patrick Kennedy. He and I had been teammates since we were ten years old, playing for Joe Russell's Angels in Little League. By high school, most pitchers knew how to throw at least three pitches: fastball, curveball, change-up. PK had all three, along with a nasty knuckleball that he had been hurling since we were ten years old. Even when they knew it was coming, all that most batters could do was close their eyes and pray their swing connected with the floating, dancing orb before it crossed the plate. Despite years together as a battery, watching PK shake off signs for other pitches until he nodded for the knuckleball signal always made me nervous.

By game time, the stands for both teams were full. My girlfriend, Ana, was still at soccer practice and my mom was at another event with my two younger brothers. Even with the early start, however, my dad was able to get out of work in time to make it, still wearing his mechanic's uniform and the grease-stained evidence of a day spent taking care of others. After the National Anthem, Dad gave me a thumbs up from the stands as I walked out for the start of the first inning. The Hurricanes' leadoff hitter approached the batter's box, and the umpire shouted what I hold as two of the most comforting words in the English language: "Play ball!"

PK made quick work of the first three Hurricane batters. Our Hornets got off to an early first inning lead by PK helping himself with a two-run homerun. The score was two to zero at the end of the first inning.

For the next several innings, our teams went back and forth. For my two at-bats, I hit two singles without scoring, after a double play in one inning and a force-out by infield fly rule in another. Entering the seventh inning, the score was two to one, and the Hurricanes were making a comeback.

The Hurricanes' catcher started the top of the seventh off with a single to left field. I shouted "Turn two" to the infielders, hoping to get the next batter to hit a ground ball for an easy double play. I called for a fastball down and in, and the batter chopped a one-hopper to our third baseman who had trouble fielding it. He did not attempt a double play, and instead threw across the infield to first base with the runner beating the throw by a step. No outs, a double play still in effect, PK followed with two strikeouts, which brought a pinch hitter to the plate with two outs and Hurricane runners on first and second. Our coach called time-out and walked to the mound, a bad move I thought, which interrupted PK's rhythm. PK and I talked coach out of bringing in a reliever, and I returned to my place behind the plate. Before squatting down, I shouted "Two down, look alive!"

First pitch, ball inside. Second pitch, a called strike. Third pitch, a curveball that was fouled off. Fourth pitch, another curveball that started down the middle of the plate instead of inside and hung a split second too long and then, "Crack!" A line drive to right-center field, gathered up on one hop by our outfielder. I checked the lead runner who was already rounding third base by the time the center fielder was delivering his throw. Everyone was screaming "Four, four, four!" demanding the throw to home plate, but I knew it wouldn't arrive in time. As the incoming throw skipped on the grass behind the pitcher's mound, I took a step and a half forward to give the baserunner a clear path to the plate.

A quick glance up the third baseline and in slow motion, out of the corner of my eye, I caught a glimpse of the baserunner launching himself toward me with both legs extended. There was no chance of avoiding a violent take-out slide. First feet, then shins, then the entire body weight of the baserunner came crashing down into my left leg.

Upon impact, I collapsed to my left, folding on top of myself like a hinge, feeling my anterior cruciate and medial collateral ligaments tear apart. The pain was so extreme that I passed out, waking to the most blood-curdling scream I had ever heard. Someone was badly injured.

Who was it? Did he need my help? It was me.

I opened my eyes, turned my head to the left, and saw my left cleat up near my left shoulder. Legs don't bend that way, I thought. The baserunner was standing over me, afraid at what he'd done. With years behind the plate himself, he knew it was a dirty play. I shouted, "I gave you the plate!" And just as the first sound of his voice started to crack in response, I heard my dad shout, "Get the fuck away from him!" To this day, it was the first and only time in my life I had ever heard my dad use that word. This was serious.

Lying there on the baseball diamond, covered in clay and sweat, I was terrified that my baseball career was over.

My dad and my teammates carried me from the field and loaded me into the brown Ford Econoline van that PK's father always parked behind the home team dugout. Mr. Kennedy was a career postal worker in Winter Park who, for as long as I can remember, finished his route in time to throw batting practice for one of the many teams that PK and I played on together. As a batter, I tended to crowd the plate and Mr. Kennedy had a penchant for throwing inside and plunking me if I ever started to get too many hits off him. He never apologized, but he always gave me a wink as if to say he was helping to toughen me up or build my character. His wink was an endearing Irish gesture which served its purpose on this day when every ounce of toughness was needed.

To stabilize my leg, Mr. Kennedy emptied one of the 5-gallon buckets filled with baseballs into the floor of the van and propped it behind my knee. My dad slid a canvas bat bag behind my back for me to lean against.

As he slid the door shut, my dad told me "You'll be okay. I will call Dr. Zink and meet you at the hospital."

I already knew this doctor –William P. Zink, M.D. – because two years prior he took care of my youngest brother, Joel, when he broke his ankle in a skateboard injury. It happened around the time of Joel's tenth birthday and was followed by several months of him in a plaster cast, receiving physical therapy while the bones healed. Joel's x-rays showed two bones being held together by a screw that Dr. Zink had surgically inserted into his growth plate. I remember that this impressed me as an example of a real-life medical miracle.

The doctor was a well-known pediatric orthopedic specialist who, in addition to being recognized as a highly skilled surgeon, had a good reputation for treating children with severe cases of hip dysplasia both in Orlando and on medical mission trips in Guatemala. He was in his early forties, a father of two young children. His wife managed his medical practice, along with a grandmotherly office assistant named Hazel. He felt familiar to me. He had an easy smile, wore a bow tie, and referred to us as "youngsters." I liked him. I trusted him.

After arriving and being admitted to Winter Park Memorial Hospital, Dr. Zink visited me in preparation for arthroscopic surgery on my left knee the following day. It was late, on a weeknight. I remember thinking that I was inconveniencing this man during the evening when he should have been home with his wife and two small children. I was grateful for the special attention he was giving me.

I spent the night in the hospital, still covered in sweat and clay dirt despite my mom's assistance with the "rinse free" shampoo the hospital provided. Ana and her sister visited. It was the first time that our young love was interrupted by a serious illness or injury where one of us was the focus of the hallway chatter between nurses and doctors. I could not make out the details of what they were saying, but the tone sounded serious. Ana looked nervous, perhaps about something she overheard on her way in. I did not possess the emotional maturity at the time to say so, but I was scared.

The next morning, on February 14, 1990, Dr. Zink performed surgery to repair my torn anterior cruciate and medial collateral ligaments. I remember waking up in the recovery room, my mouth extremely dry. A sweet nurse commented that I probably felt like I had a "mouthful of shit-kickers camp out on your tongue," and gave me water. Shortly afterward, Dr. Zink visited me in the recovery room and scheduled a follow-up appointment to be held in his downtown Orlando office within the week.

At the follow-up, post-operative appointment, Dr. Zink evaluated the fiberglass cast on my left leg and recommended it be recast because it had wrinkled during setting creating an uneven, rough edge that rubbed the top of my inner thigh. Dr. Zink slid my shorts down, looked, and remarked that the irritation would be fixed by the new cast. He rolled me on my side to examine the back of my leg, and after placing his body between me and my father who was seated in the corner, the doctor inserted his ungloved finger into my rectum. I was startled. Then, after pulling my shorts up, as he rotated my body back to a prone position, he ran his fingers along the inside of my waistband and reached to touch my genitals. It was quick, but definitely not the same type of touch that I had experienced before during a routine sports physical: no direction to turn my head and cough, just his ungloved hand holding my testicles.

I know my father did not see this, for two reasons that I can remember. First, if there was one thing that my father never tolerated, it was harmful language or acts toward his children. Second, with a house full of boy athletes, joking about the hernia exam in a regular sports physical was commonplace. Teasing reminders to turn our heads and never cough in a doctor's face as he felt your testicles during the hernia exam always got a laugh. My father did not tell this joke then nor afterward related to any visit where he accompanied me to see this doctor.

I was terrified. I was also utterly confused as I wondered why the doctor was doing something that no other doctor had ever done to me. It was both clinical and something else – not sexual, but sex-like, but only because I had no other context to associate that type of touch with. And I could not figure out why he was doing this when he was seeing me for a knee injury.

At the time, I was 16 years old and, like most boys my age, was moving through life with a peacock strut and a near visceral repulsion to all that seemed or felt "gay." I knew I faced several months of healing and rehabilitation ahead of me, and I began to worry that he might do this again to me at my next appointment. What if he did? Who would I tell? Given Dr. Zink's reputation in the community, who in the hell would believe me? What would my teammates say?

I could still remember, with white-hot intensity, the public humiliation that one of my eighth-grade teammates endured when a fellow classmate dropped by his house on the walk to the bus unannounced and caught him masturbating before school. A pubescent conch's call from "the discoverer" summoned an otherwise like-minded mob of boys – who were probably jacking off on their own sometime during the prior 24 hours – to his lawn.

"Faggot" they shouted, despite the interrupted yet solitary act. "Homo" they teased, ignoring the fact that the boy's girlfriend was on board the school bus they had just missed.

I could still remember what it felt like to sit at the cafeteria table and listen to the scintillating details of this savage suburban story recounted by our own versions of Ralph and Simon and Piggy, where facts and figures about sex and sexuality gave way to sensationalism and zero-sum self-preservation.

I could still remember what it felt like when "the masturbator" walked into the football locker room for the first time after spending two weeks at home to recover from the self-harm of tearing his own braces off to avoid further humiliation at school. We all whispered, some snickered, yet nobody offered solace or comfort.

If this is what happens to a boy caught in a natural act, albeit in an embarrassing manner, what would happen to me if the details of another man fondling my balls or putting his finger in my ass got out? I was embarrassed and afraid.

As a result, I didn't tell anyone. Looking back, I wish I did. I had no idea just how much worse it would get.

3

Exposed and Ashamed

Following my initial post-operative appointment in February 1990, and through September 1991, when I left for college, I visited Dr. Zink's office for numerous follow-up appointments to monitor the healing of my knee and the progress of my physical therapy. At the time, the standard protocol for repairing partial tears of the medial collateral and anterior cruciate ligaments of a young athlete like me was to brace the leg for a period of six non-weight-bearing weeks.

During the initial two-weeks of recovery, because of the awkward size and weight of the full-length fiberglass cast, I stayed home to learn how to walk with crutches rather than immediately return to school. When the hard cast was removed and replaced with a soft foam and Velcro alternative with a titanium joint that could be set at various angles to promote flexibility, I returned to classes and began a daily after-school regimen of outpatient physical therapy.

In the torturous month that followed, each day's one-hour treatment regimen began with twenty minutes of lying prone while a physical therapist held my foot, unlocked the joint of my knee brace, and slowly bent my lower leg toward my buttocks in a motion that produced a chicken-bone-and-cartilage crackling sound that belongs in a nightmare. Tough, teenage boy tears blurred my vision for the remaining forty minutes, which were split between electronic muscle-stimulation and an ice bath.

Eventually, I was allowed to walk, then swim, then run, and eventually lift weights. By the fall of 1990, when I was able to return to playing football and eventually baseball in the spring, I would go to Dr. Zink's office to review the fit of various knee braces. Some were better than others, but all earned me the nickname "Robo-Pick" from my beloved linebacker coach and school guidance counselor, Phil Richard.

At each appointment, most of which I attended on my own as I was driving by then, Dr. Zink repeated the same acts of sexual assault and molestation as he had before. Whatever the purpose of my office visit, before my appointment ended, Dr. Zink would have me lay on his examination table, roll me onto my side and insert an ungloved finger into my rectum. He would then fondle my genitals, as he had done since my first post-operative visit. Each time, he seemed to take more and more time to finish. I remember leaving each one of these visits feeling nauseous and lightheaded immediately afterwards. Sometimes, I remember feeling like I was in a fog. I had difficulty concentrating.

I specifically remember the difficulty with concentration because it was at the same time I was enrolled in an SAT preparation course that met twice each week at Rollins College along with a couple of high school classmates. Rollins College and its idyllic campus had always been a place of comfort for me. It is where I learned to swim, to waterski, to play piano, and where my grandfather earned his master's degree in business administration from the Crummer Graduate School of Management. It is where I first learned of the tradition of Fox Day that began with President Hugh McKean in 1956 and was resurrected by President Thad Seymour when I was a young boy. It was an officially-sanctioned day of hooky that granted students an unscheduled day off in the spring. It was a fun memory of an otherwise hallowed institution that was appropriated by many more Winter Parkers than were enrolled as students. It was a place that always felt comforting, but at this time in my life it did not.

On most of these SAT prep course days, I would go home with my friend Jennifer Hannigan after school and then get dropped off with her in the evening for class. We were kindred spirits, both of us athletes with similar knee injuries. Neither of us were very excited about studying for the SAT, but we enjoyed spending time together.

On the other SAT prep course days, instead of going home to an afternoon study session at Jenn's house before our class at Rollins, I would drive myself to Dr. Zink's office for a follow up appointment immediately after school.

Turn left out of Bishop Moore High School campus and drive south on Edgewater Drive toward my father's alma mater, Edgewater High School. Turn left on Par Avenue, pass Dubsdread Golf Course and merge onto Interstate 4. Drive south on I-4, bumper to bumper traffic, through downtown Orlando, exit at Gore Street and jog several streets to the east and south to arrive at 61 W. Columbia Street.

After checking in with the office assistant at the front desk, I would eventually be taken to an examination room. On several occasions at these follow up appointments, without a parent or guardian present, Dr. Zink would ask me to go into a room in the back of his office for a procedure he called a "Moire."

According to medical literature, Moire topography is a procedure used for school screening of scoliosis. The device resembles a rectangular windowpane, and the photographs taken through the device display patterns that show contour lines of the body that appear similar to those on a relief map.

For my Moire procedures, I recall that as I entered the room, Dr. Zink would turn off the overhead lights and turn on a spotlight. He would direct me to remove my clothes and stand behind the Moire device while he shined the spotlight in my eyes. I was unable to see him as he spoke in a quiet voice and told me to lower my underwear as he took photographs. I remember feeling uncomfortable.

In the same quiet voice, the doctor instructed me to lower my underwear further until my pubic hair showed. He took more photographs. "Please lower your underwear further," he said again. My penis was almost exposed. He took more photographs. I felt very embarrassed. "Lower your underwear further," he said again. I followed his instructions, exposing my penis and testicles. He took more photographs. By this point, I felt scared and panicked.

Among the things I remember finding particularly strange about these experiences was that photographs of other boys undergoing the same procedure were tacked to the walls. Other similar photographs were laying in boxes scattered around the floor. I could never make out the faces in the photographs, but it appeared that there were dozens of different boys who had been photographed in the same way that I had.

Each session lasted for what felt like an eternity before the doctor finished and told me to get dressed. I could not wait to pull my underwear back up, put my clothes on, get out of the room, into my car and drive for what was the comfort of friends, the order of advanced math formulas, the rhyme and meter of reading comprehension passages, the Rollins College campus.

I remember sitting in class, in a seat that Jenn had saved for me, listening to the instructor deliver a lesson in what sounded like a muffled foreign language, and then feeling my heart race, my breath get short, and the most terrifying feeling: Panic.

Panic – because of something dreadful that happened to me just hours before that I could not tell anyone about.

Panic – because of something so humiliating that someone did to me during the afternoon before class that I could not get out of my mind.

Panic – because of something that felt so uncomfortable and foreign that it disrupted my normal confidence and natural sense of myself.

Panic – because of something so frightening as a pitch-black room filled with pictures of naked boys who had all been exactly where I was without anyone knowing and without ever being saved.

Normally, I followed right along, but on these evenings my brain was useless. On these evenings, the purpose of an SAT exam felt futile. With my high school graduation around the corner, I was taking this course and studying extra hard to get into college, to start a path toward medical school and a career in sports medicine. But right now, what good would an SAT prep course do for a kid who was going to die? At least, that's how I felt on these evenings when the familiar smell of oak and books and chalk dust betrayed me, leaving me alone in a room full of people who would never know the fear I was feeling.

4
Viaje de Compañeros

After graduation from Bishop Moore High School, in the summer of 1991, I volunteered for Viaje de Compañeros, a program that brought recent high school graduates from the Diocese of Orlando, Florida, to live and work in the Diocese of San Juan de la Maguana, Dominican Republic. The purpose of this program was to immerse ourselves in a cultural exchange while establishing an understanding of the principles and practices of liberation theology and social justice.

My viaje or "trip"was facilitated by being paired with a Dominican family who hosted my visit and served as my companion during my stay. Because of an intensive schedule of preparation, my knowledge of the Dominican Republic, its history, and politics was strong. My familiarity with its people, language, and culture was limited, however. This was a world that bore no resemblance to my home community.

The pueblito I was assigned to is named Pedro Santana. It sits high in the mountains, on the Rio Artibonito, which runs along the border between Haiti and the Dominican Republic. It is one of the most remote places on the island of Hispaniola, and the poorest island in the western hemisphere.

As morning broke, throughout the day and into the night it was not uncommon to hear the phrase "no hay agua" or "no hay luz" spoken by husbands to wives, mothers to children, or children to the gringo occupying the full-size mattress covered in mosquito netting in the room adjacent to the dirt-floor sitting room.

No disappointment that there was no running water to bathe, to do dishes, to clean clothes or to cook in. Simply no hay agua - there is no water.

No frustration that there was no electricity to shine a light in the dark, to keep refrigerated food safe to eat, to power a household appliance that might make life simpler. Simply no hay luz - there is no light.

Most days, my morning started under the mango tree seated at a wooden table outside the house my Dominican family shared with me. A breakfast of a simple, non-perishable version of café con leche and a roll, followed by a walk to la iglesia to meet the rest of the compañeros. Meeting at the church was not necessarily to attend mass. The church building was at the center of Pedro Santana. It was one of the only buildings made of stone with a concrete floor, a solid roof, and enough seats for everyone in town. The church, however, had no pastor and no regular worship schedule. For now, we were the church.

Unlike many faith-based, summer missions, Viaje de Compañeros was not a work trip. Sure, our group of recent high school graduates were involved in a variety of community service projects to help improve certain aspects of community life in Pedro Santana. We freshened up public buildings with new coats of paint for the church and school buildings. We gave the local library a make-over. We worked from house-to-house installing basic water filtration systems made from two ten-gallon plastic buckets, a carbon filter, and a spicket, that strained pollutants from the river and well water used by village residents in their homes. But the real purpose of our immersion experience was to get to know the individuals and families who resided in our sister diocese, and to gain a perspective on what life is like in one of the poorest countries in our world.

Before these experiences, I had never given much thought to the phrase "less fortunate" that was often used to describe people in far-away lands who did not have the basic essentials needed to sustain life. In my mind, it was a code word for people who deserved my charity because they were simply unlucky. The idea, however, that so many of the Dominicans I had befriended during my visits had the same bad luck all at the same time did not sit right with me.

In my mind, the phrase "less fortunate" gave me comfort knowing that there was always another hand to be dealt that could include better cards . . . pocket aces, a full house, or a royal flush. As my time in the Dominican Republic ended, however, I was starting to realize that my Dominican friends were playing with a different set of house rules. During that summer I was slowly beginning to understand just how little depends on chance for people like my Dominican friends and other marginalized people at home and around the world. The choices of others have as much to do with their lot in life as their own self-determination. If I believed my Dominican friends should have what they need to simply live, what changes did I need to make in my own life to live more simply? If I thought that my Dominican friends deserved to live in peace – and not peaceful submission – was I willing to work for justice to help make that possible? It would be a long time before I had the maturity and insight to fully understand the paradox I was living in, but something had begun to change in me.

After returning from my viaje, I spent the last few weeks of summer working for my father in his auto repair shop. My girlfriend and I had broken up as the prospect of maintaining a relationship with me in college and her as a high school senior seemed unworkable. Friends were already starting to leave for college.

During those last few weeks of summer in Orlando before leaving for college myself, my participation in social activities were becoming more difficult. I skipped several going-away parties, excusing myself for not feeling well. A trip to my primary care doctor ruled out parasites from the water I drank in the Dominican Republic. It did not, however, explain my insomnia or the fever dreams that were waking me in the middle of the night.

"No, nothing specific," I told Dr. Joseph Covelli when he asked about the details of my dreams. He never learned that these nightmares were variations of a scenario filled with images of being stuck in a sweltering hot, pitch-black room, alone with Dr. Zink.

Perhaps it was the unmooring from the safe harbor of family and friends that disrupted my psyche and pushed these images to the surface. All I wanted to do was to drown them and erase them from my mind. Drinking heavily usually did the trick – mostly fortified wine or cheap bourbon copped from the local liquor store for the cost of an extra bottle for the random adult carpenter, painter, or landscaper I hustled as they sought the same solace. However temporary, booze was my cure.

As summer came to an end and college was approaching, I began having pain in my hips and leg. My mother encouraged me to make an appointment with Dr. Zink before leaving for college. Perhaps there was something that he could do or prescribe to help alleviate the pain, she suggested, unaware of the abuse I had been enduring. His only opening was for the Saturday morning I was scheduled to leave for college. While it was uncommon for a doctor to see a patient on the weekend, Zink was different. He had always been eager to make himself available.

I was reluctant to follow my mother's suggestion to take the Saturday opening that Dr. Zink offered me. I could have made up an excuse about needing to leave a day earlier for college. I also could have lied and told my mom and dad that my leg was feeling better. I was nowhere near ready to tell my parents about the things Dr. Zink had been doing to me over the previous18 months, so after a simple calculus that this would likely be the last time that I ever saw him, I called his office and scheduled my visit.

On Saturday, the day of my appointment and of my departure for the University of South Florida in Tampa, I waved goodbye to my family

22

from the driveway. There were not many tears, as I planned to drive back the following weekend with my best friend and college roommate, Mike Moran, to gather the rest of our belongings for the semester.

I drove away, taking the back way through Audubon Park past the old naval air station, Glenridge Junior High, and the T.G. Lee Dairy. Zink's office parking lot was empty when I arrived, and I remember wondering if I had the appointment date and time wrong. His office door was open, however, and he greeted me when I walked in.

As usual, Zink did his thing. He examined my legs and my hips. He put his ungloved finger in my rectum. He fondled my genitals. He told me that he wanted to take more photographs.

Before walking me to the back of the office where photographs were taken, Dr. Zink handed me a small plastic cup. It contained a liquid that he told me would help with my pain. I drank the liquid, tossed the cup into the trash can and walked inside the darkened room.

The room spun. I collapsed, face down on the floor. I could feel the low-pile carpet on my face. I could see the pictures of other naked boys tacked to the walls and spilling out of boxes on the floor. I could hear something, maybe someone, in the room. The whirring of a fan, the shuffling of feet, the click of a lock, and the jangle of a belt buckle. I tried to get up, but I could not move.

Then something terrible happened. An unspeakable violation of all that I was. I tried to scream and tell him "No!" I could not stop the rape.

Instead, I buried it. Then, life took over.

5
The Spark

By the following summer, in 1992, between my freshman and sophomore years of college, I had volunteered to be a mission trip leader
with Viaje de Compañeros. I looked forward to returning to the
Dominican Republic.

I was particularly looking forward to seeing Wilson and Enrique
again. I got to know both boys the previous summer. Born in Pedro Santana, they had lived their entire lives in wooden clapboard houses that
were less that a minute's walk apart on the last street in the northwest
corner of the town before the steep decline of the riverbank. Wilson was
the oldest of five children and lived with his single father. Enrique had a
younger sister, and lived with his mother, father, and abuela. Like many
13-year-old boys, Wilson and Enrique loved baseball and the salsa and
merengue music of Juan Luis Guerrera and his band, Cuatro Cuarenta.

The previous summer, Wilson and Enrique were regular companions
on our day trips into the Dominican and Haitian countryside. Together,
we had ridden in the back of a camioneta to visit the local sulfur caves,
regarded by many as a natural healing destination. On another trip, we
crossed the puente over the Rio Artibonito into Haiti, to visit the local
goat market. On another, we hiked to the cave of St. Francis of Assisi,
where locals claim – inaccurately by about 5,000 miles – St. Francis was
born. By the time I returned to Pedro Santana in the summer of 1992,
both boys had grown several inches in height and had started shaving.
They still loved baseball, and salsa and merengue, but girls had now
been added to their list of interests.

One day, the camioneta we had arranged to give our group a ride
back from a work project installing bucket-based water filtration devices
in a group of homes on the town's outskirts did not show up. The day
was getting late, so we decided to make the four-mile walk back into
Pedro Santana. The late afternoon sun was sweltering hot, and the
walk was miserable. It was nearing the end of our viaje and many of the

compañeros were homesick and ready to return to their families and the comforts of home in the United States.

As we arrived in town, I noticed that the local bodega was open. Apparently, the power was on for the day, which meant that there was a possibility of cold sodas in the cooler. The gringos in our group lined up and each took a soda from the cooler, popped the top, and proceeded to drain the contents of each glass bottle within minutes. I did, too. We said our goodbyes, and all dispersed to go to our individual homes scattered throughout the town.

When Wilson, Enrique, and I arrived at our house, the two boys called out for their younger siblings. They had a surprise. As the children gathered, I finally realized what their excitement was about. By then, my cold soda was a distant memory, but these two 13-year-old boys were still holding theirs. As their younger brothers and sisters gathered, the boys offered each one a sip. Smiles spread across the young children's faces, as each one offered their own version of "muchas gracias."

On a scorching afternoon, this small act of kindness and generosity by two 13-year-old Dominican boys, best friends, ignited a spark in me. It has burned ever since.

Where did two boys who live in one of the poorest towns in the entire Western hemisphere learn to be so selfless? What inspired their generosity? Is this a habit that came naturally to them, or was it something they were taught? How might I follow their example, and could I use my own experience to inspire others to develop and practice similar habits of generosity?

These questions were with me as I began my sophomore year of college. I was still well on my way toward pursuing a pre-medicine degree, working through the required biology, chemistry, physics, and mathematics courses. By the end of the academic year, however, my career ambition of becoming an orthopedic surgeon and serving my community by fixing broken athletes was starting to fade.

No – not fade, but drift. Unmoored and separated by a betrayal of my understanding that all doctors swore an oath to do no harm, pushed along by a hope that I might find another way to demonstrate the finest tradition of this calling, I began to doubt.

Until this point in my life, the aspiration of becoming a doctor was terra firma in my mind. It was a certainty, an absolute, a commitment to pursuing a helping profession to which I felt anchored to – in part because of my own curiosity, interest, and ambition. In part because of the esteem I held for my childhood doctors.

I can still picture their faces. A cloud of witnesses to the young man I was becoming and to the course I was following. A Hippocratic totem that signaled safety, security, and no harm.

Dr. Luis Spinelli was my childhood pediatrician whose drop-every-thing mentality excused hasty departures from social gatherings – and even Mass – whenever patients called. Someone whose booming voice and thick Argentinian accent vanquished my pinprick fears I had when the time came for back-to-school vaccinations, and someone whose untimely death from a heart-attack at age of 63 left the world a little less decent and kind.

Dr. Joseph Covelli was my childhood pulmonologist whose familiar demeanor combined with a "fuggetaboutit" swagger let his patients know that he was in control and that you were going to be okay. His attention and careful administration of medicine rescued me from asthmatic suffocation on more than one occasion.

Dr. Robert Thornton was my childhood neurologist whose genteel manner and seersucker confidence exemplified the kind of success and personal satisfaction that comes with a commitment to excellence in a profession.

Drifting out to sea, unknowingly, it was these faces, with all their care, comfort, and encouragement, that gave way to the face of a creature from the deep that I had never imagined: lurking, hungry, and ready to strike as it had done so many times before.

6

Past is Prologue, Doctor Accused of Misconduct, February 6, 1994

In the fall of 1993, I made the bittersweet decision to change majors to study political science and Spanish. I was 20 years old, and while I was still interested in a career helping others, I decided it was going to be doing something other than by following my childhood dream of a career in sports medicine. I felt good about this plan and for having the courage to follow a new path.

Making this change brought new focus and energy for my last two years of college and my post-graduation plans. I had a rigorous schedule mapped out for my junior year at the University of South Florida in Tampa, followed by summer classes with sociologist, educator and social justice advocate, Dennis Kalob, at Loyola University in New Orleans.

My senior year would be spent in San Jose, Costa Rica, splitting my time between earning course credit for a Spanish minor by attending language school and working in an internship for a human rights attorney affiliated with the Oscar Arias Foundation and the Inter-American Court of Human Rights during the week. Weekends were spent chasing waves.

Each Monday through Thursday morning began with a bus ride along the Inter-American Highway from the apartment Mike Moran and I rented in the suburban neighborhood of Curridabat to the capital of San Jose. Morning classes were followed by a lunch of gallo pinto con huevo revuelto – a Costa Rican businessman's plate of rice, beans and herbs blended and cooked together, topped with a scrambled egg, and served with a simple cabbage slaw and copious amounts of Salsa Lizano.

The last few hours of each afternoon continued with a shuttle-race between the law office, the law library, and the Court to assist with the preparation of an amicus curiae brief being filed in a case against the

27

government of Nicaragua for the crime of homicide against the minor Jean-Paul Genie-Lacayo.

On October 28, 1990, this 16-year-old boy drove to his home in a subdivision of Managua and attempted to pass a convoy transporting military personnel, which included several members of the escort guard of General Humberto Ortega. The boy's car was machine-gunned with more than 50 rounds of ammunition and, according to witness testimony, left on the side of the road with the dead boy inside. An investigation by the Nicaraguan authorities resulted in no arrests for the murder of Genie-Lacayo, nor for the murder of several witnesses. My small contribution to this case, seemingly insignificant at the time, eventually resulted in a judgement against Nicaragua which included reparations to the boy's family. It was a glimpse of the greater good I would pursue in my future vocation.

After graduation, but before attending graduate school, I would dedicate a year of my life to voluntary service as a lay missioner working among homeless men and women in New York City. As I progressed on my journey, my parents were supportive. So were many of the other adults in my life who I relied on for guidance and support for most of the big decisions I made.

One of the strongest affirmations came from my childhood confirmation sponsor and longtime surfing buddy, Dr. John Guarneri. I remember telling him about my plans, and in return, receiving a copy of the following speech often attributed to Archbishop Oscar Romero with a handwritten note in the corner that read: "Jeff, Thought you would enjoy this as you proceed on your journey. Dr. G." It is one of my most prized possessions.

It helps, now and then, to step back and take the long view.

The kingdom is not only beyond our efforts, it is even beyond our vision.

We accomplish in our lifetime only a tiny fraction of the magnificent enterprise that is God's work.

Nothing we do is complete, which is a way of saying that the kingdom always lies beyond us.

No statement says all that could be said.

No prayer fully expresses our faith.

No confession brings perfection.

No pastoral visit brings wholeness.

No program accomplishes the church's mission.

No set of goals and objectives includes everything.

This is what we are about:

We plant seeds that one day will grow. We water seeds already planted, knowing that they hold future promise.

We lay foundations that will need further development.

We provide yeast that produces far beyond our capabilities.

We cannot do everything, and there is a sense of liberation in realizing that.

This enables us to do something, and to do it very well.

It may be incomplete, but it is a beginning, a step along the way, an opportunity for the Lord's grace to enter and do the rest.

We may never see the end results, but that is the difference between the master builder and the worker.

We are workers, not master builders; ministers, not messiahs.

We are prophets of a future not our own.

What I did not know in late 1993, as I began this vocational transformation, was that at the same time, back in my hometown, several young boys were showing their own courage by speaking up for themselves. They had come together, with help from the Orlando District Attorney, to pursue criminal charges and expose a serial child sex abuser who they knew and trusted. He was their doctor.

Surprisingly, this was not the first time this doctor faced similar charges. In 1990, Dr. William P. Zink, who treated patients at Orlando Regional Medical Center and Florida Hospital Orlando (now doing business as AdventHealth), was indicted and eventually cleared of criminal charges in 1992 after a judge ruled evidence against him had been obtained with a faulty search warrant.

Despite being cleared from the 1992 criminal charges, however, an administrative complaint of sexual misconduct would be filed with the Florida Board of Medicine, the State's top medical regulator. This administrative complaint was eventually reviewed by the Board of Medicine in 1994.

In Florida, complaints and reports involving health care practitioners like Zink who are licensed by the State are investigated for the Board of Medicine by the Department of Health to determine if related Florida Statutes have been violated. Actions that may be taken are administrative in nature and can result in a reprimand, fine, restriction of practice, remedial education, administrative expense, probation, license suspension, or license revocation.

Title XXXII of Florida Law pertains to the regulation of professions and occupations. Chapter 458 pertains to medical practice. Section 458.329, the Florida Statute listed in the complaints, pertains to "Sexual misconduct in the practice of medicine." It reads as follows:

The physician-patient relationship is founded on mutual trust. Sexual misconduct in the practice of medicine means violation of the physician-patient relationship through which the physician uses said relationship to induce or attempt to induce the patient to engage, or to engage or attempt to engage the patient, in sexual activity outside the scope of the practice or the scope of generally accepted examination or treatment of the patient. Sexual misconduct in the practice of medicine is prohibited.

The administrative complaint associated with the 1992 criminal case began with the standard legal form identifying the petitioner, in this case the Florida Department of Health, the respondent, Dr. William P. Zink, a licensed physician in the state of Florida with a last known address of 61 West Columbia Street, #8, Orlando, Florida 32806, and the Florida Statute pertinent to the complaint.

In the original complaint, facts were included describing violations of this Florida Statute involving three patients. Patient 1 was a 13-year-old male who began seeing Dr. Zink for an injury to his left ankle on or about November 9, 1988. Patient 1 was diagnosed with a fibular fracture and was placed in a short-leg cast which was subsequently removed on or about November 30, 1988. The following March, Patient 1 returned to Dr. Zink for an examination of this injury, at which time clinical photographs were recommended. At an office visit on April 1, 1989, Dr. Zink took more than 100 photographs of Patient 1, all of which were in the nude and in various positions. These included multiple nude photographs with Patient 1's legs spread and anus exposed.

Patient 2 was a 15-year-old male who first saw Dr. Zink on or about September 15, 1989, with complaints of pain in his right knee and leg. The diagnosis was a probable benign cortical defect, and a computerized scan confirmed no malignancy. On or about October 30, 1989, Dr. Zink obtained a moire and took more than 100 photographs of Patient 2, all of which were in the nude and in various positions. These included multiple nude photographs with Patient 2's legs spread and anus and genitals exposed. According to the complaint, several of these photographs were of Patient 2 in a "supine position with his legs spread, as viewed from below, exposing his genitals and anus."

Patient 3 was a 14-year-old male who presented to Dr. Zink on or about August 31, 1988, with a fractured left ring finger and a fractured left femur. After surgery and an uneventful recovery, on or about November 19, 1988, Dr. Zink obtained a moire and took photographs of Patient 3 to show range of motion and alignment of his lower extremities. Of the multiple moire images taken, however, all were nude images of Patient 3's torso that did not show leg length. As for the photographs, more than 100 were taken of Patient 3 in the nude, including several taken from behind showing Patient 3 with his legs spread.

In an amendment to the original complaint, an additional patient ("Patient 4") was included for the Board of Medicine to consider in its deliberation. On or about June 18, 1991, Patient 4, a 13-year-old male, visited Dr. Zink for a pre-surgical physical in advance of the removal of an ingrown toenail. According to the amended complaint, although Patient 4's medical history did not warrant it, Dr. Zink performed a rectal examination. This rectal examination "lasted approximately one minute, without any other adult in the room."

When the administrative meeting of the Board of Medicine concluded, a final order was issued resulting in Zink's license receiving a reprimand. In addition, Zink was ordered to have a patient's parent or a licensed nurse present during all examinations and clinical photography sessions. Zink would be required to maintain a contract with the Physician Resource Network (PRN), a program for treating impaired professionals. Zink would be prohibited from using rectal examinations or clinical photography in the practice of medicine until authorized to do so by PRN. He would pay a $25,000 fine. Finally, Zink's license to practice medicine would be placed on a three-year probation which, among other things, required direct supervision by a monitoring physician, quarterly reports, and performance of 200 hours of community service per year.

Going forward, the Board prohibited the 43-year-old Zink from taking photographs of patients or performing rectal exams until mental health counselors determined he could do so. Even then, the Board issued a clear order that he may never do those things to children without a parent present.

In his defense, Dr. Zink said he had done nothing wrong. "On the basis of this misunderstanding with one patient, a cascade of misinterpretation has arisen," he said.

Seated between his wife and his attorney, Skip Dalton, Zink explained that the photographs, for which he did not charge, helped him document patient progress. He said rectal exams were a standard part of surgery preparation.

Comments from some Board members, however, did not seem to agree. One of the Board members who expressed serious concern was Cecile Scoon, an alumnus of Harvard University, the University of Virginia Law School, and the United States Air Force JAG Corps. "I don't know if you are in denial, or what here," she said to Zink. "In my opinion, you have covered up your interest in children, specifically your interest in boys, with your professional ability."

As for the perspective of the pediatric patients who filed the complaint, one mother expressed her disappointment saying, "I don't think this is strong enough. He shouldn't have anything to do with children."

For the time being, that would seem to be a possibility. Zink's attorney said that it could be some time before he returned to work. Because of yet another new complaint being filed, Zink had been ordered to temporarily stop practicing medicine and obtain counseling.

Although these events transpired in a pre-internet world, they would quickly become the talk of the town. For a community that had so closely aligned itself with Walt Disney World as "the happiest place on earth," the headlines that would follow in the local newspaper were an embarrassment and a sign that evil still lurked in Orlando's shadows.

Zink was not a sinister villain, nor a cackling witch, rather, a serial child sex abuser disguised as a children's doctor, hiding in plain sight.

7

Past is Prologue, Doctor Put in Jail After New Fondling Complaint, February 19, 1994

D eep in the heart of Texas, there once was a place where perverted doctors accused of inappropriate conduct with patients were sent to receive treatment as a condition of maintaining their medical license. Sometime in the early part of 1994, Dr. William P. Zink had gone there, likely following the advice of his lawyer.

Since 1960, when Plano was a little farming town of thirty-five hundred people on a flat terrain dotted with barbed wire, sheep, and scorpions, the community had grown to an industrial and commercial backlot technoburb north of Dallas. The now defunct hospital was one of a few facilities nationwide that operated what Florida Statute 456.076 defines an impaired practitioner program.

According to the statute, an impaired practitioner program is "one that is established by the department of health to contract with one or more consultants to serve impaired or potentially impaired practitioners for the protection of the health, safety, and welfare of the public." It is a clever euphemism that does not distinguish between the most common reasons professionals are referred, such as alcohol and drug dependency and other mental health and psychiatric reasons, or pedophilia.

It is possible that Zink's decision to go to the Texas program was related to conditions imposed by the Florida Board of Medicine linked to the1990 indictment on charges that he took nude photographs of eight young boys from 1983 through 1989. Prosecutors eventually dropped the case in 1992, after a judge disallowed key evidence citing a faulty search warrant. Specifically, and rather unbelievably in hindsight, the judge sided with the defense attorney's "use a scalpel not a sledgehammer" position that the search warrant was violated because the seizure of evidence from Zink's office comingled nude photos and medical records of the eight boys represented in the indictment with records of dozens of other unnamed victims. Reprobate legal tactics aside, a crisis of a public trial and a potential criminal conviction was averted for the time being, but apparently not the depraved impulse.

It is not clear if Zink's admission to the impaired practitioner program was for alcohol or drug dependency, an underlying mental health or psychiatric reason, or a last-ditch effort to expunge a hard-wired penchant for young boys. What is clear, however, is that it was at this Texas facility where Zink was arrested and taken into custody on Thursday, February 17, 1994. He was held without bail while awaiting extradition to Orlando, where he would face possible criminal charges related to new accusations that he molested a 12-year-old male patient who he treated for foot problems more than 30 times between 1989 and as recently as January 13, 1994. The new charges related to this complaint are sexual battery on a child younger than 12, lewd acts upon a child, and use of a child in a sexual performance.

Arrests such as this were not uncommon in this town. Home to 150,000 hard-working, family-oriented residents, it was this community where just six months before Zink's arrest, seven-year-old Ashley Estell was taken from the playground adjacent to the soccer complex where her ten-year-old brother was playing in the annual Labor Day tournament. Rumors of child molesters swirled among parents. Police found Ashley's body days later in a nearby field. She had been strangled.

When authorities finally arrested little Ashley's killer, several community members recognized him as a participant in one of the searches organized to help find her. Public outrage followed when it was discovered that, at the time of Ashley's murder, her killer was "mistakenly" out on parole after serving just eighteen months of a ten-year prison sentence for a 1988 crime of breaking into a Dallas home and touching the breasts of an eleven-year-old girl. Apparently, the parole board erred by reviewing a file that only mentioned the burglary conviction. A convicted child molester was set free, only to prey on an innocent child again.

While waiting for his extradition, Zink's defense attorney, Kirk Kirconnell, was quick to publicize the news that no formal charges had been filed by the state's attorney, no fire to see here. There was, however, plenty of smoke.

According to police reports in this new complaint, the 12-year-old boy's mother told police that Zink had given her son 15 rectal examinations without a glove and had fondled his genitals about 25 times. His mother told police she or the boy's father were present during the examinations, but Zink always stood between them and the child.

34

She also told police Zink took dozens of nude pictures of her son in various poses, including with his legs spread. She said she was in the examining room but thought Zink's actions were an acceptable procedure.

The woman told police she became suspicious when Zink called on New Year's Eve, saying the boy needed a pre-operative exam before his January 5 foot surgery. Records show the child already had the exam on December 27. She said the doctor was alone when she brought her son to Zink's office on a Sunday.

Her son told police Zink handled his genitals and photographed him nude during that visit. After the surgery, the mother told police she and her son visited Zink's office for a follow-up exam. During the exam, the mother said she saw Zink put his hand down the front of her son's pants.

After being contacted by the mother, police served a search warrant on Zink's office and seized dozens of photographs. Orlando Police Detective Frank Roche said that two independent medical experts labeled the photographs pornography.

As troubling as this one case is, it is not the only matter related to Dr. Zink that Orlando police would be working on. Detective Roche asked prosecutors to file additional charges in four other cases following complaints that Zink fondled the genitals of two 4-year-old boys and a 12-year-old patient, now 18, and that he performed a rectal exam on a different 13-year-old boy before surgery for an ingrown toenail.

"If any of these charges are filed, we will defend them and defend them vigorously," attorney Kirkconnell said to the Orlando Sentinel. "These charges all have to do with interpretation of the way he practices medicine. Medicine is an art as well as a science. You are going to have a difference of opinion. Dr. Zink is disappointed about the new accusations but is eager to return to Florida as quickly as possible to fight them."

As a defense attorney, Kirk Kirconnell made a career out of convincing juries of how easy it is for the average person, without specialized training, to misinterpret the actions of a skilled practitioner. Of course, a rectal or a genital exam might seem uncomfortable to an observer, but science would back his client's claim that these were necessary procedures. Yes, nude photographs of children might seem repugnant, but not when you hear testimony of how these pioneering techniques are used and the transformative results they help patients achieve.

What, then, can be said for the letter written in January by eight medical residents from Orlando Regional Medical Center ("ORMC") expressing concern about the way Dr. Zink examined children? Among the examples given in the letter, which was forwarded to state medical regulators by hospital administration, was an observation by two residents that they saw Zink improperly touch a boy's genitals after the doctor finished placing a cast around his hip and leg.

What does a mother who works in the bakery of the local grocery store know about pre-operative procedures? And what does a father who works as a house painter know about medical photography? What do eight medical residents know about what is and what is not appropriate when examining children?

Zink knows. He knows pediatric orthopedic medicine. He knows what to look for when examining photographs of children's bodies, the curves of their limbs, the contours of their torsos. He knows how to touch children during a medical exam, how to place his hands in ways that soothe his patients, make them feel healed. Surely, these are just differences of opinion.

8

Past is Prologue, A Mother Deposed, June 23, 1994

On the morning of June 23, 1994, a mother of three boys who were all treated by Dr. Zink for various sports-related injuries arrived at the State Attorney's Office at 250 North Orange Avenue a little after 8:30am. She arrived an hour early in order to have time to find the room where a deposition was scheduled in the case of the State of Florida vs. William P. Zink. Even with the help of her youngest son, a 16-year-old rising junior and football star at the local Catholic high school, she was concerned that an inherited retinal condition would make it difficult for her to navigate around the darkened hallways of the building.

When she arrived at Room 423-B, the mother was greeted by attorney Dennis Quintana, another one of Zink's lawyers who would be attending the deposition. After offering the son a seat in the hallway and a bottle of water, Quintana directed the mother into the small conference room where she was introduced to Eve Russ, the electronic court reporter for the Ninth Judicial Circuit and the attorney who would be conducting the deposition.

In a southern drawl, Willie May introduced himself as Assistant State Attorney and told the mother that he would be taking her deposition on behalf of the plaintiff in the criminal case against Dr. William P. Zink. After she was sworn in, May began by asking the mother to state her name and address for the record.

"Are you employed outside the home?" May asked.

"Yes, I am. I am a Registered Nurse and work at (REDACTED) Hospital," the mother answered.

"And how long have you been a registered nurse?" May asked.

"Since 1971, for 20 some odd years working full-time, mostly in critical care," the mother answered.

"Did you ever work in orthopedics?" May asked.

"Yes," she answered. "From 1977 until around 1980."

"Do you know William Zink?" May continued.

"Yes, I do. I have three sons and he's treated all of them for orthopedic injuries," she answered.

"Your name has been listed as a witness that the defense says they intend to call at the trial, so I have a few questions for you in that vein." May continued. "You said that your sons have been treated, over the years, by William Zink. Have you been present for any of those examinations that were conducted?"

"Yes, I have," the mother answered.

"In any of those examinations, were photographs taken by William Zink?"

"Yes, they were."

"In any of those photographs, were the children completely naked?"

"Yes, they were."

"In any of those photographs, were the genitals or penises of the children revealed?"

"Yes, they were," the mother replied.

"Then, I think it might be helpful to – well, let me ask another – couple of general questions first. In any of the examinations that you were present for, when William Zink examined any of your sons, did William Zink conduct a rectal examination?"

"No, he did not," the mother answered.

"In any of the examinations for which you were present, did William Zink touch or manipulate the penises or genitals of your sons?"

"Yes," she answered.

"What is your youngest son's name?"

"(REDACTED)," the mother answered.

"And for what conditions did he see William Zink?"

"He saw him for – initially, for a fractured ankle. And then, he saw him for various knee problems, sprained ankles, back and – I don't recall the others," the mother said.

"Were photographs taken by William Zink on all the occasions when (REDACTED) saw him?"

"Not on all the occasions, no," the mother answered.

"Given that you're a registered nurse and, in fact, have worked in orthopedics at certain times in your career, do you know why it is that photographs were taken for treatment of these kinds of injuries?"

"Yes, I do," she answered.

"Why?" May asked.

"Dr. Zink explained to me, with (REDACTED) – he had a fracture at the epiphyseal or the growth plate of his ankle, and it was at a critical growth period of his life, he was ten – that this could affect the growth of his leg. Dr. Zink said that this injury could make him shorter, so he would have to be carefully watched because of where the injury was."

"Dr. Zink explained to me he was going to do clinical photographs on (REDACTED) to watch the progress of his leg lengths and his hip lengths. I don't fully understand exactly where the growth difference was, but he said that he would be showing me and would be really observing the length because there could be some discrepancy because of where the injury was."

"All right. Did you ever see any of the photographs that Dr. Zink took of (REDACTED)?"

"Yes, I did," the mother answered.

"Okay. Now, your next oldest son: his name?"

"The middle is (REDACTED)," she answered.

"Oldest is (REDACTED), right? Middle is (REDACTED). Youngest is . . .?" May paused.

"(REDACTED)," the mother answered.

"(REDACTED). That's who's outside?"

"Um-hum," she confirmed.

"For what purposes did (REDACTED) see William Zink?"

"Let's see. (REDACTED) I believe initially saw him for an ankle, then saw him for a hip fracture, and then saw him for a knee injury," the mother answered.

"From approximately what age to what age did (REDACTED) see William Zink as a patient," May asked.

"Oh, goodness. Probably – I can't really recall, but I – they were all soccer related injuries and he played all four years of high school on the varsity team. So he was probably 15 – I'd say 14 or 15, but I'm not really sure when he first saw him," she replied.

"Were you present when (REDACTED) saw William Zink for examinations on all occasions?"

"My husband or I," she said.

"On those occasions when you were present for examinations by William Zink, did he conduct any rectal exams on (REDACTED)?"

"No, he did not."

"On any of the occasions, when you were present for exams by William Zink, did he ever touch or manipulate (REDACTED)'s penis or genitals?"

"No, he did not."

"Did William Zink take any photographs of (REDACTED)?"

"He did not do clinicals on (REDACTED)," the mother answered. "He did moires on (REDACTED)."

"Were you present for some of those?"

"I was not present – I was in the building. I was not present in the room," the mother answered.

"Did (REDACTED) have moires taken, also?" May asked.

"Yes, he did."

"Did (REDACTED) ever report to you that William Zink had touched his penis or his genital area?"

"No, he did not," she answered.

"Did he ever report that William Zink had conducted any rectal exam upon him?"

"No, he did not."

"Same questions as to (REDACTED), did he ever advise you of any such event?"

"No, he did not."

"Now the oldest is (REDACTED). For what purpose did (REDACTED) see William Zink?"

"He saw him for minor injuries, ankle, shoulder. But he saw him for a major knee injury, and that was in 19 . . . I think '89 or '90, when he had a major knee injury," the mother answered.

"About what age was (REDACTED) when he saw him?"

"(REDACTED) was a junior in high school. So I'm thinking he was 16 or 17. He was probably 16.

"More soccer injuries?" May asked.

"A different sport," the mother clarified.

"Oh. Good," said May. "I was concerned there. I had heard that soccer was such a good game: however, it looks like it has its violent side too."

"No. I guess."

"And were you present for the occasions when (REDACTED) was examined by William Zink?

"Yes, I was."

"Did William Zink conduct any rectal exams on (REDACTED)?"

"No, he did not."

"Did you ever see William Zink touch (REDACTED) penis or genitals?"

ANSWER MISSING FROM THE DEPOSITION.

"Did William Zink take any photographs of (REDACTED)?"

"He did moires on (REDACTED)," mother answered. "I'm not sure about clinicals, but I do know he did moires on (REDACTED) because he also saw him for scoliosis. All three boys have scoliosis. It was picked up at one point or another during the boys' sports physicals."

At this point in the deposition, the mother was starting to feel tired. Remembering all the details of the medical histories of three active boys who were all involved in various competitive sports was difficult.

"This was all, you know, over a long period of time so I'm a little confused as to which son received which. But I know that Dr. Zink did moires on (REDACTED), but I am not sure about clinicals."

Sensing the mother's fatigue and slight frustration, May changed the focus of his questions. Now that he had a good understanding of the numerous ways in which Dr. Zink had interacted with the mother and her three young boys as patients, May wanted to get a better sense for how she felt about him since his arrest.

"Have you talked to William Zink since he was arrested on these charges?"

"No, I - let's see. Talked to him, no, I have not," the mother answered. "I did receive letters."

"So he has written to you, but you haven't written to him?"

"To the family. To the family."

"To the family. Have you read those letters that William Zink sent to you?"

"Yes, I have."

"In any of those letters, did William Zink make any statements or comments about whether or not he had committed any of the offenses with which he is charged?"

"No, he did not."

May wondered whether the mother had kept the letters that Dr. Zink had written her from jail? If she kept them, would she let May read them? He suspected not but made a mental note to discuss pursuing the idea with his colleagues at the DA's office.

Either way, he was starting to get a sense of Zink's personality. Dr. Zink was a skilled and highly sought-after pediatric orthopedic surgeon, but his rather feeble appearance and yielding demeanor belied the typical alpha archetype. He preyed on athletes but lacked physical prowess to overpower them, so he adapted and found more subtle ways to manipulate his victims. Powerful narcotics were at his disposal.

From his professional reputation, years of volunteer service caring for children in need, and the character witness statements that were already collected in preparation for trial, Zink appeared to have a conscience. A psychopath? No, but he was just as calculating. He knew what he did to these young boys was wrong. His letters to their parents were repentance, disguised as familiar correspondence. Instead of asking for absolution, however, he simply included a return address. When the mothers and fathers of his victims wrote back in reply, he was washed clean.

May continued with his questioning.

"Have you made any contribution to a defense fund for William Zink?"

"No, I have not."

"Has your family or anyone you know of?"

"No."

"Okay. When was the last time that you saw William Zink, as best you can recall?"

"We attended one of the bond hearings, and that's the last time we saw him," she answered.

"Have you offered your support to William Zink in any fashion since he was charged with these offenses?"

"Emotional support to the family to -- to Joan -- the family has written a couple of letters to him."

"Do you know of Mrs. Zink -- of William Zink's wife as well?"

"I do know Joan, um-hum."

"Do you know her on a personal basis?"

"From being in the office so many years, we've come to know her."

"I have one final question," May said. "Do you have an opinion on what the reputation of William Zink is, in the community among others, as opposed to what you personally think?"

The mother told May that she couldn't comment on Dr. Zink's reputation among others. "I only know how I feel and my family feels."

"I have no further questions," May said and he ended the deposition.

Looking back on this mother's testimony, I wonder why Zink's attorney, Kirk Kirconnell, would never call her to testify in his client's defense?

She was a registered nurse who seemed to understand and felt comfortable with the clinical explanation that Dr. Zink provided for the purpose of taking nude clinical photographs and moires of her own children. She was an attentive parent, who gave a sworn deposition stating that, except for that first visit with her youngest son, she had never observed nor received a report from any of her three children that Dr. Zink manipulated their penises or genitals. Similarly, she had never observed nor received a report that rectal exams were performed. She was a regular visitor to Dr. Zink's office, who was familiar with Dr. Zink's wife and wrote supportive letters to his family while his client was in jail awaiting trial.

If the jury would not believe this mother as a character witness in Zink's defense, I am not certain who they might believe.

If Kirkconnell were around today, I might ask him these questions. He died, however, in 2012 at the age of 69, carrying the answers to his grave.

Perhaps someday I will find the courage to ask the mother. I know her, after all. I am her oldest son.

9

Past is Prologue, Zink Goes to Trial on Molesting Charges, June 27, 1994

Unbeknownst to me, ten days following my twenty-first birthday, and five weeks into my summer classes at Loyola University in New Orleans, jury selection was beginning at the start of the trial of William P. Zink in state circuit court in Orlando, Florida. Unlike 1992, when similar charges against him were dropped before a trial, this time a jury would be asked to determine whether Zink molested children under the guise of medical care, or if he was being persecuted unfairly for his medical techniques.

Felony or difference of opinion?

Police and prosecutors said that Zink used his trusted position to satisfy his sexual urges for young boys. The 43-year-old doctor was being charged with molesting five boys between 1987 and 1993, and with taking explicit photos of one of these patients and another boy. If convicted, Zink faced up to 27 years in prison under state sentencing guidelines, and possibly more if requested by the prosecutor.

The burden of proof would fall on the shoulders of veteran sex crimes prosecutor, Robin Wilkinson, who would have to convince a jury that the acts that Zink performed on his pediatric patients were lewd. She would also have to prove the same of the thousands of nude photographs of young boys seized from Zink's office by police.

Arguing against her and the criminal charges brought against his client, attorney Kirk Kirkconnell would contend that Dr. Zink's care of his patients was of the highest quality both medically and ethically. He and his legal team would use information collected during pretrial questioning and court testimony to discredit the six boys accusing Zink of sexual assault and molestation in this trial brought by the State of Florida.

They had already succeeded in getting one of the charges dropped. One of the accusers, a 12-year-old boy, corrected his prior statement to police that Dr. Zink penetrated his anus during 15 ungloved rectal examinations given to him. Instead, the boy told Kirconnell and his team of lawyers in a pretrial interview, that Zink had only touched but not penetrated his anus. As a result, Zink would not be tried for sexual battery, avoiding a possible life prison sentence, and was instead freed on $50,000 bail.

By the time the trial began before Orange County Circuit Judge Alice Blackwell White, dozens of upstanding supporters had come forward to help Dr. Zink fight against what many portrayed as a police vendetta and an opportunistic financial gain for his accusers.

One of these supporters was Tricia Madden, a lawyer and friend of Zink's whose son visited the doctor for almost 10 years to cure "walking" troubles. In an interview with the Orlando Sentinel, she said, "I think if justice prevails, Bill will come out acquitted. I don't see anything he's done except practice good medicine."

Another supporter was Becky Dreisbach, a fellow church member and Zink's neighbor. She told the Orlando Sentinel that the trial would be "the most unjust thing for a man to have to defend his name in this way for being such a wonderful person."

What was it about Zink that made it so difficult for so many people in the Orlando community to believe that a man capable of good deeds can also been capable of molestation?

Discussion about crimes against children and their consequences are documented in public records and historical texts dating back to the beginning of civilization. Many of these instances involved perpetrators who were known by many as upstanding members of society, only to be discovered and, in many cases, convicted for the most repugnant criminal acts beyond imagination. In fact, in the months leading up to Zink's trial, federal legislation pertaining to these exact legal issues was making its way to President Clinton's desk for signature and would ultimately become law as the Jacob Wetterling Crimes Against Children and Sexually Violent Offender Registration Act ("Jacob Wetterling Act").

The Jacob Wetterling Act is a United States law that requires states to implement a sex offender and crimes against children registry. It is named for Jacob Wetterling, a Minnesota eleven-year-old who was abducted by a stranger in 1989 and was missing for almost 27 years until his death was confirmed when his remains were found in 2016. The strength of the law comes from tying federal block grant eligibility to specific requirements for states to annually verify the addresses of sex offenders and sexually violent predators.

Monsters like those that prompted the Jacob Wetterling Act have always been lurking in plain sight, going about their business without drawing attention only to strike when opportunity presents itself. The subsequent Meghan's Law, enacted in 1996 to strengthen the Jacob Wetterling Act has shown us that. Meghan's Law is named for seven-year-old Megan Kanka, a New Jersey girl who was raped and killed by a known registered sex offender who had moved into a home across the street without her family's knowledge. The law requires states to publicize the information collected through the requirements of the Jacob Wetterling Act to provide communities with more opportunity to keep children safe from sexual offenders.

By the time of his 1994 trial, Zink had been practicing medicine in Orlando for more than a decade. Records show that by this time he had treated more than 10,000 patients. Eight of those patients who he treated between 1983 and 1989 had already come forward in 1990 with charges that Zink had taken sexually explicit photographs of them. While the case was eventually dismissed due to a technicality – a faulty search warrant – the pall of suspicion around Zink had already been cast. Yet, somehow otherwise sound-minded members of the community – a registered nurse, an attorney, a realtor, and fellow church member – could not bring themselves to believe that he was capable of the acts that he was being accused of committing.

Still, somehow, a total of 14 boys were standing up for themselves, enduring what were likely some of the most uncomfortable and embarrassing conversations of their lives: talking about traumatic experiences that would likely scar them forever, fighting their own monster.

Their Jabberwock and its eyes of flames,
Their Dracula and his bloody fangs,
Their Werewolf and its fearsome howl,
Their old yellow dog and his rabid growl.
In front of parents,
a judge,
police detectives.
Surely, now, they would be protected.

10

Past is Prologue, Zink Patient "I Thought That's What He Was Supposed to Do." July 6, 1994

The morning's proceedings began with the testimony of the youngest of the six boys being represented by the State's Attorney's Office as plaintiffs in the criminal trial of William P. Zink. A key prosecution witness, the boy would undergo rigorous questioning today by defense lawyers.

In January, the boy had been interviewed by Orlando police. He told them then that his pediatric orthopedic surgeon, William P. Zink, had performed 15 ungloved rectal examinations during several medical appointments over the previous five years. As a result, Zink was charged with sexually battery and faced a life sentence if convicted. After a lengthy deposition with lawyers in June, however, the boy recanted partly, stating that Zink had only penetrated his rectum once. After the deposition, prosecutors dropped the sexual battery charges, deciding to proceed with other charges that could still result in a sentence of 27 years in prison if Zink was convicted.

Because of the boy's age and the anticipated sensitivity of his testimony, Judge Alice Blackwell White limited attendance in the courtroom to the witness's family, attorneys, court workers, and the media. Zink's wife, Joan, and his brother-in-law were also allowed to observe, as the second week of the trial began.

The 12-year-old Orlando boy fidgeted and yawned as he took the stand. Sunburned cheeks and sleepy eyes suggested he was tired, perhaps from a long weekend of swimming and watching fireworks in celebration of Independence Day.

Prompted by Assistant State's Attorney, Robin Wilkinson, the boy told the jury that his orthopedic surgeon fondled his genitals about two

46

dozen times during medical appointments to help him correct problems with his feet and legs that made it difficult for him to walk. Specifically, the boy said that Zink conducted nude examinations in which he touched his testicles, penis, and anus. During one of the exams, the boy said that Zink put an ungloved finger inside his rectum.

The boy also described being photographed in the nude by Zink during multiple visits to his office over a five-year period. He said he was taken to a back room in Zink's office and posed so that the doctor could take photographs of his genitals.

"I thought that's what he was supposed to do," the embarrassed boy testified, "... 'cause he's a doctor."

The boy told the jury he feels better now that he no longer receives treatment from the popular Orlando pediatric orthopedist.

The defense attorneys were quick to dispute the boy's testimony, saying no rectal exams occurred. They also argued that at least one of the boy's parents was present for all exams that were all done for medical purposes.

Zink's attorney's suggested that the Orlando police misinterpreted the boy's description of what had happened to him. The police, however, disagreed. Assistant State's Attorney Wilkinson suggested that if there was anything confusing about the boy's deposition, it was likely due to his extreme discomfort in the way he was questioned by Zink's defense attorney. Wilkinson went on to tell Judge Blackwell that during the boy's deposition, defense attorney Jim Russ touched the back of the boy's body on or near his buttocks while questioning him about Zink's past medical examinations of him.

At the request of prosecutor Robin Wilkinson, Orange Circuit Judge Alice Blackwell White ordered defense lawyers not to touch the boy or hover over him during his testimony.

"That would be intimidating to an adult, much less a 12-year-old," Wilkinson told the judge.

A man's freedom was on the line, and Zink's defense attorneys were pulling out all the stops to sway the jury's opinion in favor of their client. Certainly, everyone accused of a crime is entitled to competent counsel. I wonder if Zink believed that he was getting what he was paying for? With at least one more day of testimony scheduled in his trial before jury deliberation, Zink would have to wait to find out.

11

Past is Prologue, Dr. Zink Gets More Medical Criticism, July 9, 1994

An Orlando pediatric orthopedist didn't need to perform rectal exams, touch children's genitals, or take nude photographs of them to treat their ailments.

On July 9, 1994, this is what Dr. Charles Price, director of pediatric orthopedics at Orlando Regional Medical Center, told the jury presiding in the trial Dr. William Zink. At the time of his testimony, Dr. Price was already recognized as an expert in the field of pediatric orthopedics.

Since giving his testimony in 1994, Dr. Price has continued to practice medicine in Orlando, and has contributed substantially to the field of pediatric orthopedics both clinically and academically. He has trained numerous fellows and residents in the appropriate orthopedic care of children and is known internationally and nationally for his leadership of several prestigious pediatric orthopedic medical societies. Dr. Price has published more than 100 manuscripts, book chapters, and textbooks on pediatric orthopedic medicine, with countless references in the medical literature to his expertise on the treatment of hip dysplasia in children. He is also a professor of orthopedic surgery at the University of Central Florida Medical School.

Therefore, when Dr. Price told jurors that Dr. Zink could have allowed children to wear underwear for photographs, he was speaking as an expert who had treated hundreds of patients. His assertion that there was no medical reason to feel some boys' genitals when they visited for foot and leg troubles was an experienced point of view.

Zink's defense lawyers disagreed. Instead of denying these acts took place, attorney Roy "Skip" Dalton argued that all of Zink's actions were routine and done for medical reasons. Dalton was a graduate of the University of Florida Levin College of Law. His private practice spanned nearly three decades before serving as counsel to United States Senator

Mel Martinez. He was eventually appointed by President Barack Obama and confirmed by the United States Senate as a judge in the United States District Court in Florida's middle district.

Dalton must have had to swallow hard to proclaim the following:

Putting an ungloved finger in the rectum of a 12-year-old boy fifteen times. Routine and medically necessary.

Touching the penis and testicles of a 12-year-old boy twenty-five times. Routine and medically necessary.

Taking more than 100 nude photos of a 12-year-old boy with his legs spread and anus exposed. Routine and medically necessary.

Furthermore, to discredit Dr. Price, attorney Dalton suggested that Price's testimony disagreeing with Zink's methods stemmed from a challenging history between the two doctors who were once partners but who did not part amicably. He also suggested that Price's opinions about nudity in patient photography were personal standards rather than medical, and that Zink's methods were simply more thorough than those of Price.

I imagine Dalton, now a father and grandfather, might have a different opinion today. Would he want the same "thorough" methods applied during medical exams of his own loved ones? I would hope not, but that is not what appears to have been the case 17 years later in 2011 when asked by the United States Senate Judiciary Committee to describe the ten most significant litigated matters which he personally handled. Proudly listed at number two is the case of Florida v. Zink, in which Dalton served as co-counsel and is on record stating that multiple ungloved rectal examinations, fondling, and nude photographs of a 12-year-old boy by a doctor were "routine and medically necessary."

The trial proceeded slowly, and at one point, a defense attorney tested the patience of state Circuit Judge Alice Blackwell White. After clearing the courtroom, the Judge berated the lawyer for his inappropriate conduct, essentially bullying one of the child witnesses as he gave his testimony. Media were given strict orders not to publicize the names or faces of any of the witnesses or jurors, out of concern that peer pressure would influence decisions in such a high-profile trial.

Surprisingly, Zink remained rather calm throughout the proceedings. His affect was almost as if he was medicated or sedated. Throughout the trial, the College Park father of two sat among his three lawyers, often consulting with them quietly. His wife, Joan, who would eventually go on to be his practice administrator, sat directly behind him.

The verdict would come soon.

12

Past is Prologue, Jury Clears Zink of All Charges of Molestation, July 27, 1994

The morning of July 26, 1994, the air outside the downtown Orlando courthouse hung heavy, a few hours ahead of thunderstorms forecast for later in the day. After several weeks, the jury in the trial of the State of Florida versus William P. Zink would deliver its verdict today.

"All rise," the bailiff barked as Judge Alice Blackwell took her seat at the bench. The courtroom was filled with supporters of the plaintiffs and the defendant to listen to a verdict that could mean justice for six boys and a long prison sentence for the Orlando pediatric orthopedist charged with sexually assaulting and molesting them under the guise of medicine.

Judge Blackwell reminded the court and those in attendance of the decorum, and then turned to the jury's foreman to ask if a verdict had been reached. The jury of three men and three women had deliberated 13 hours over two days before reaching the verdict.

"Yes, a verdict has been reached, your honor," the foreman answered.

"Please proceed," Judge Blackwell instructed.

"For the charges of lewd acts upon a child, we find the defendant not guilty."

"For the charges of use of a child in a sexual performance, we find the defendant not guilty."

"For the charges of possessing material depicting sexual performance by a child, we find the defendant not guilty."

Amid the gasps and cries of the six boys and their supporters, Judge Blackwell gaveled the trial closed and told the defendant that he was free to leave.

The 43-year-old defendant smiled with relief, flashing the same gap-toothed grin from my first appointment. In plain view of the six boys who he was accused of sexually assaulting and molesting, he hugged and thanked each of his attorneys, their unpleasant assignment now complete. He then turned for a long embrace with his wife, Joan, who sat behind him throughout the four-week trial in Orlando.

Accompanied by his attorneys, Zink left the courtroom quickly. He did not want to speak with the media. He walked from the Orange County Courthouse in the driving rain. Instead, attorney Kirk Kirconnell spoke on his behalf.

"He is grateful the trial is over and the judicial system works the way it is supposed to," Kirconnell said. "The verdict says what we've always maintained: Dr. Zink is a caring, gifted physician and a good, moral man."

While some of the six victims expressed anger at the decision, they said they would accept the verdict and move on with their lives. Others said they believed the justice system had failed.

"I'm in shock. He should not have gotten off scot-free," said the grandmother of a 4-year-old boy who said she saw Zink hold her grandson's genitals for several minutes during a visit for problems with a leg brace.

"I'd just like to see him (Zink) get some help. He's a good surgeon and doctor. His morals ... he's just not right."

The grandmother of Zink's main accuser – a 12-year-old boy who said Zink repeatedly pulled back the foreskin of his penis and ran his finger around his anus – said her grandson had hoped Zink would not be allowed to treat any more patients. The boy had visited for five years for walking troubles.

"If he keeps on practicing, he will need a nurse definitely beside him," the grandmother said. "He really has a problem."

As for the jury's decision, one of the jurors said that they ultimately agreed that Zink's exams and nude photographs had legitimate medical purposes. Other than the testimony of the boys, there was no concrete evidence Zink acted lewdly while treating patients.

"We did not feel there was any evidence to support it was done with lewd intent. We can't assume what he was thinking when he was doing it," said the juror, Jerry, who agreed to an interview with the Orlando Sentinel on the condition that his last name be withheld.

"I think what it came down to was we had a lot of conflicting testimony."

Jerry said most jurors appeared at the start of the deliberations to have an idea of how the case would go. He said they analyzed every piece of evidence and reviewed their notes, debating important points of each case one at a time.

Although it was not part of their role as jurors, they felt it would be helpful in the end to send Zink a message, Jerry said.

First, Zink should generally stop taking nude pictures of patients, he said. Although Jerry said jurors agreed that the pictures played an important role in patient care, it should be clear that society's values are changing, and many people don't approve of nude pictures of children.

Jerry, who works in entertainment productions, said jurors relied on experts who said Zink's photos, and nude photos in general, were medically acceptable. He said jurors compared them with similar photographs in medical textbooks that defense lawyers provided.

Jurors also believed the photos depicted mostly the same poses over time, which Zink explained was necessary to chart patient progress. Prosecutors had contended the poses – on the floor with legs spread and genitals exposed – were varied and that pictures could have been taken with children wearing underwear.

Second, jurors suggested Zink should make more of an effort to communicate with patients about what he is doing. His accusers complained that he gave no reason for touching genitals or requesting that clothing be removed for photos. Defense attorneys claimed patients jumped to conclusions about what happened because they didn't understand.

Jerry said jurors considered the fact that Zink's accusers didn't immediately object to his medical procedures. Parents were often in the room but said they didn't question Zink because they believed he was an authority. Jerry said it appeared accusers's memories weren't entirely reliable.

"Dr. Zink looked like a very focused person to us. He probably just had a lack of communication with patients to put them at ease," Jerry said. "Dr. Zink needs a little better bedside manner in communicating with patients."

I imagine Zink's response to hearing these messages from the jury after dodging nearly 30 years in prison.

Ok, Jerry. I've got it. No more taking nude photos of kids in my office. Given all this attention, I imagine there might be some additional scrutiny to those procedures going forward, so I'll figure something else out. In fact, I recently heard about this new, wonderful invention called the internet. In a few years, I bet I could simply type the words "nude pictures of boys" into a computer and find exactly what I need, completely out of sight from anyone.

And yes, Jerry, I agree. Better communication with my patients. Telling a boy before putting an ungloved finger in his rectum or before I hold his penis and testicles should put him at ease.

A sip of liquid medicine might put another boy patient of mine at ease too. Good thing I have ample access to the strongest narcotics on the market. I'll do anything to help this muscular, athletic youngster to relax and put him at ease.

Put him at ease, hmm. I like the sound of that, Jerry.

13
Awakening

Sometimes I wonder if I had been aware of Zink's trial when it was taking place in 1994 or if I had been involved with the prosecution, whether the outcome would have been any different. Would it have affected the lives of those boys or the course of my own life in a different way?

During the summer of 1994, the countdown for the launch toward a newfound vocation in a helping profession had begun. I do not believe it is fair to put the burden of the idea that I might have made more of a difference if I were aware of or at Zink's trial on myself. All the oxygen in my life then was being consumed in this white-hot combustion that put me on a hypersonic path in the opposite direction, far away from whatever pain my attendance at the trial might have brought on.

After graduating from college in 1995 and spending a year of volunteer service as a lay missioner working among homeless men and women in New York City, I enrolled in graduate school at the University of San Diego School of Education and Leadership Studies to pursue a master's degree. My studies included conducting two participatory action research projects among disparate, but similarly marginalized populations: Hmong refugees engaged in the creation of a cooperative preschool, and teenage students on the Cathedral Catholic High School Surf Team.

Among the many insights I had about my future vocation from my time in both New York City and San Diego was the realization that I was very skilled in two essential functions of a career in philanthropy and the nonprofit sector – making money and helping people. While I do not believe I could have pursued a career in sales for a company or product I did not believe in, I had a knack for being able to construct a compelling case about an important cause and soliciting donations from generous people who trusted me and the causes I represented with their charitable investments.

54

In 1997, I moved to Chicago for my first professional job, leading a nonprofit charitable organization that provided residential medical recovery for ill and injured homeless adults discharged from the hospital. For the next ten years, I continued my career in the nonprofit sector. I married Debby, an Irish Catholic girl from Chicago's north side who was a licensed clinical social worker. The early years of our marriage took on an ethos of "us against the world," two civically minded friends with a shared commitment to social justice. This was my ground control, settling my nerves and all the frenetic energy on this launchpad.

After almost five years as newlyweds, Debby and I started a family, first with a son, Colin, and then a daughter, Olivia. We loved each other and did our best to be good for one another.

Despite Debby's clinical knowledge of and familiarity with her own genetic predisposition toward depression and substance use disorders, she would succumb to the ravages of alcoholism. I divorced her, initially to protect the children from her risky behaviors but eventually to establish a framework for the possibility of co-parenting in the future. After some time apart, the co-parenting began and it started to work, until it didn't. Alcoholism eventually took Debby's life. She was my closest friend, and the mother of my two young children. I was heartbroken and forlorn, but resolved to continue living for myself, Colin, and Olivia.

When I met Stephanie in the fall of 2008, I was a single father with two young children. She was a city-chick living in downtown Chicago, originally from Palm Springs, California. She had never been married, no children, and had recently moved to Chicago from New York City for her career in healthcare philanthropy and public affairs. Stephanie and I met as colleagues, and by early 2009, we had fallen in love. It was a bashert union that defied all calculations. We kept it very quiet at work, and nobody suspected anything. By the time we both lost our jobs the following summer, victims of the Great Recession along with dozens more colleagues, we were both relieved to finally be able to live publicly as a couple. We resolved to follow each other anywhere.

In 2010, we moved to Bakersfield, California for my work and got married. Stephanie adopted Colin and Olivia, and by June of 2013 baby Grant was a little over a month from being born. He was wanted by everyone, especially Stephanie's father, Dr. Marvin Brooks, who was in the last stage of his fight with cancer back in Stephanie's desert hometown of Palm Springs, California. I turned 40, and Marvin died at Eisenhower Medical Center, the hospital he founded in Rancho Mirage, but not before meeting Grant via ultrasound.

Despite my grief, I kept a promise to Marvin that I follow through with the birthday gift I made to myself to attend Stanford's Hasso Platner School of Design. My goal was to learn innovation and human-centered design. What I learned was the gift of empathy. Gifts are meant to be cherished, and my life was full of them.

We were happy, working hard, deeply ingrained in that Central Valley community when in early 2015, Vero Beach, Florida came calling. A significant promotion in my salary for a new community foundation CEO role and a chance at island life was ours for the taking, so we took it. The home we found on the barrier island on Florida's Treasure Coast was close enough to visit my family in Winter Park, close enough to drive to my grandmother's 90th birthday celebration, close enough to attend her funeral a few weeks later.

Nothing in those first two and a half years after returning to my home state of Florida, however, felt ominous. Until the night of October 16, 2017, I was seemingly unaware of just how close I was to the scene of my childhood sexual assault and molestation. It was as if the horrific memories were submerged more than 1,000 fathoms below the surface. No light. No sound. No movement. Complete stillness, until they were unmoored.

Sitting in our bedroom that evening in October of 2017, Stephanie and I Googled "Dr. William P. Zink" and were shocked by what we read from past stories in the Orlando Sentinel. He was charged, tried, and acquitted for the same criminal acts he committed against me, except these proceedings detailed in the news articles resulted from reports made by other boys in the Orlando area.

Even more troubling were the headshot photos of Dr. Zink from his own practice's website and from AdventHealth Orlando's website. This was the first time I had seen a photo of him since I stopped seeing him as a patient in 1991.

It was these headshot photos that were fresh in my mind a week later, on October 25, 2017, when I attended an evening reception honoring donors to a local Vero Beach charitable organization that my foundation supports. As the host rose to welcome guests, his striking resemblance to Dr. Zink caused me to panic. I knew it wasn't Zink, but the mere image triggered a visceral reaction. I broke into a cold sweat, my heart started to race, and I felt dizzy. For a moment, I thought I might be having a heart attack. I quickly left the room, went to the restroom to wash my face, and ordered an Uber to take me home.

Over the course of the next several weeks, a cycle of anxiety and depression set in like none that I had ever experienced. A visit with my 14-year-old son to his pediatrician caused a panic attack during the doctor's medical examination of a pulled back muscle. Reading coverage by Ronan Farrow in The New Yorker of sexual assault allegations against Hollywood mogul Harvey Weinstein, triggered more of the same.

The daily news reports of abuse victims of Michigan sports medicine doctor, Larry Nassar, coming forward to tell their stories broke my heart. At the same time, they felt all too familiar.

Girls and young women, many of whom were aspiring Olympic athletes, were talking for the first time of years-old experiences of sexual assault and molestation by their doctor. One account, originally reported by the IndyStar newspaper in 2016, that was recirculating in the Fall of 2017 was that of Rachel Denhollander.

In a police report, Ms. Denhollander described crimes that took place when she was 15 years old and being treated by Larry Nassar for lower back pain. Over five treatments, she said that Nassar gradually became more abusive, first massaging her genitals and then penetrating her vagina and anus with his ungloved finger and thumb. She told police that her mother was present in the exam room, but that Nassar positioned himself in such a way that only her head and back were visible.

Nassar endeared himself to these families, and used his power, his status, his technical explanations, and his sleight of hand to test the limits between the art and science of medicine so that he could fulfill his perverse sexual urges. They trusted Nassar. He was like family, they said. Most kept these stories of abuse to themselves, but some told a parent and were not believed. He bet against misunderstandings until everyone understood.

Filtering in were past reports of sexual abuse within the Roman Catholic Church: anecdotes from the criminal trial of former Penn State football coach Jerry Sandusky; a horrific story of a Kansas man who won a $100 million judgement against the Boy Scouts for the sexual abuse he endured as a boy only to take his own life when the Boy Scouts of America applied the full force of its legal power to appeal and delay payment indefinitely.

As the days and weeks progressed, I would reflect on these reports and the similarities to my own abuse. I felt extreme shame and sadness. On many occasions over the next few weeks, I cried myself to sleep. Eventually, the tearfulness and feelings of emptiness would last all day.

Little things started to bother me: a sideways glance from my oldest son, an unsolicited opinion from my daughter, a disobeyed direction from the youngest son. Some nights I couldn't sleep, and other nights I went to bed early and could barely wake up the next morning. My energy was at an all-time low. These were all feelings that I had only previously heard others describe when telling stories of clinical depression.

I was scared. I knew I needed to ask for help, but I did not know how.

In an emergency, we are taught to dial 9-1-1. In an airplane, if the cabin loses pressure, we are instructed to put on our own oxygen mask first before assisting others. In school, depending on where we live, we practice earthquake, fire, tornado, or active shooter drills. These situations are fraught with fear, yet we are told that these measures can save our lives. Repetition commits these lessons to memory so that one day, if needed, we can save ourselves.

In an emotional emergency, however, I do not think I was ever taught how to get help with my own feelings, despite how simple the solution was. Nobody ever instructed me how to overcome fears of losing control, fears of being labeled weak, or fears of wandering into the realm of mental health care.

In my career in philanthropy, I was an expert in asking other people for money to support good causes. However, I was a complete and total beginner in the act of asking for help for myself. I was aware of the extreme pain I was in, however, and knew that if I did not do something soon, that my life might be in danger.

14
Asking for Help

As the holidays approached, I started to realize that my feelings were out of my control. While I was never suicidal, I was hurting. With Stephanie's support, I sought medical help and professional counseling.

The first person I asked to help me was my primary care physician. Since childhood, I have been fortunate to receive excellent primary care from every doctor that has ever cared for me. Looking back, however, I do not recall any of my primary care doctors ever asking me about my mental health.

Maybe it is because of the general good nature and positive attitude I have always possessed. Perhaps it was the cultural influences of the post-war times when most of them received their training and began their practices. Whatever the reason, it left me ill-equipped to know who or how to ask for help with something that was affecting my health as severely as any medical condition ever had. For asthma, I used an inhaler. For cholesterol, I took a statin. For the sheer terror of panic or the crushing blow of depression I had nothing other than a general reluctance to talking about it or taking anything for it. My doctor changed my mind.

I visited my doctor's office and told her about recently remembering the repressed memory of being sexually assaulted and molested as a child by my doctor. She listened to my brief description of the abuse and my recent recollection of it. She listened to me tell her how anxious and sad I was feeling. I cried and I could see in her eyes that she wanted to help me. She said, "I am so sorry this happened to you" and "I believe you." She asked if I would be open to trying a medication that could help relieve some of the acute symptoms brought on by the emergence of these repressed memories. I agreed and thankfully felt immediate relief from the medication she prescribed. I understand that this is not always the case, but I am grateful that the treatment worked for me.

My doctor also encouraged me to talk to a therapist and to incorporate some form of meditation into my daily schedule. Fortunately, I knew of a clinical psychologist whose services were covered by my insurance plan. Her office was located down the street from my house and office, which would also make regular appointments convenient. I met with my psychologist and told her about myself and the feelings I was having related to the recent recollection of a memory of childhood sexual abuse and molestation. She listened and she also told me how sorry she was that these terrible acts happened to me. I began to attend weekly sessions that helped me to start managing my feelings and gave me an objective perspective as I processed the trauma.

Somehow, because of grace, or Stephanie's love and support, or my own willingness to let go, I was able to talk to my doctor and a therapist and ask for help. I believe my decision to do so, combined with their empathetic responses, saved my life, and set me on a path that would eventually help me to overcome the despair I was feeling.

15
Taking Action

Out of concern for my own well-being and that of others who may have experienced similar unreported acts of what I believed were sexual assault and molestation, at the age of 44, I finally decided that I needed to take action.

If for nothing else, I needed to do something for myself to feel something different other than anxiety, depression, fear, or anger. If Zink was still practicing . . . still doing his thing . . . I was not going to stand by and settle for being one of his victims. I was going to fight back.

While I could not believe that I was the only victim of Dr. Zink, the absence of any public information about him or his crimes since those 1994 news articles was puzzling to me. Was I the only person whose repressed memories of childhood sexual assault and molestation were triggered by the developing #MeToo stories? Would I be the first person to speak up about Dr. Zink's criminal past since those boys at the trial? If so, given the cultural moment we were in, surely justice would be swift, and Dr. Zink would finally get what he deserved.

Perhaps it was my naivete, or simply my blind faith in a justice system that I had never really needed, which made me feel hopeful that my story would result in some measure of justice for me. In my mind, I pictured myself reporting this years-old crime, being taken seriously enough that someone would stop whatever they were doing and immediately get started on my case. I imagined Zink being arrested and finally getting what he deserved, to rot in prison and then burn in hell.

I would soon learn, however, that a history of sexual abuse among males is more common than one might think. Additionally, men are generally less likely to disclose these experiences, and when they do it is usually decades after the abuse occurred. The likelihood of Zink being punished for his crimes was extremely low and knowing this made me furious.

As I began taking action, I learned that sexual abuse of boys is more

61

common that I knew, disturbingly more common.

According to the organization 1in6.org, research shows that at least one out of every six men have experienced sexual abuse or assault, whether in childhood or as adults. Numerous studies confirm these findings, the latest of which was completed in 2005 by the U.S. Centers for Disease Control on San Diego Kaiser Permanente HMO members. The study found that 16 percent of male patients were sexually abused by the age of 18.

I was a statistic. To have a chance at justice, I would need to bring my statistic to life. I would need to find my story and tell it.

I would also have to do so in a manner where the time since my abuse would not become an impediment to my efforts to seek and obtain justice.

As I continued taking action, I discovered that reports of sexual abuse of boys often take years to surface. Sometimes they never surface at all.

According to Child USA, the national think tank for child protection, the average age for a victim of childhood sexual abuse to disclose is 52, with the median age of 48. The reasons for the delay are specific to each individual, but often involve disabilities that result from the trauma, feelings of shame and embarrassment, and even fear that a disclosure might be too painful for a parent or guardian to bear ... especially if the parent or guardian facilitated the initial or ongoing interaction with an abuser such as a priest, a doctor or a coach.

As I began to make my own plan for taking action, I started to understand that prosecuting sex abuse crimes against children is difficult due to statutes of limitations. This is perhaps the most infuriating lesson I learned.

Child USA explains that when a victim does disclose, there are two paths to justice for children who have been sexually abused: criminal prosecution and civil lawsuit. In many states, there are also administrative actions that may be taken against a doctor's medical license. Unfortunately, most child sex abuse victims who cannot prosecute, pursue administrative action with their state's board of medicine, or file civil lawsuits because they missed the arbitrary procedural deadline – the statute of limitations ("SOLs") for their claims. Most victims miss the statute of limitations because of the disclosure delay that is common among child sex abuse victims.

In my case, I simply did not remember the abuse until almost 30 years after it happened. When I did, the memories were clear but fragmented, so it took me some time to piece them all together. Once I understood what had happened to me, it took me even more time to believe how it happened. I wasn't a baby or a child, I was an athletic teenager capable of defending myself. The man who abused me wasn't a stranger, and it did not happen in some back alley. He was my doctor, and it happened in his office. Some of what he did was hidden from my parents's view, but other things were explained as routine medical procedures. At the time of the abuse, we all believed him.

The first action I took in the fall of 2017 was to pursue criminal justice. I started by contacting law enforcement. I called the Orlando Police Department and said that I wanted to report being sexually assaulted by my doctor in 1990 and 1991. My heart was pounding.

The operator asked for the address where the crime occurred, which I had to look up. I told her it was in my doctor's office at 61 W. Columbia Street, Orlando, Florida, and she asked if that was still his office. I had to look that up too and learned that his office was now in a different location at 2909 N. Orange Avenue, Suite 102, Orlando, Florida. This would require me to call a different phone number, she said. She transferred me to a detective's voicemail, and I left a message with the details of my assault.

Days later, when the detective returned my phone call, I learned that the acts committed against me did not qualify as first-degree sexual battery, for which there are no criminal statute of limitations. According to Florida law, "sexual battery" is defined as "oral, anal, or vaginal penetration by, or union with, the sexual organ of another or the anal or vaginal penetration by any other object." As a lesser offense, in my case, the definition of sexual battery under Florida law presented complications for me to proceed due to the doctor's prior claims that his acts fell within a clause in the definition that exempts acts that "were done for a bona fide medical purpose."

Even without the medical designation, however, the criminal statute of limitations for lesser degrees of sexual battery and lewd molestation against children between the ages of 16 to 18 years old would have required a report to law enforcement within 72 hours of the crime for my 2017 claim to be valid. Otherwise, the criminal statute of limitations is three years from the time of the crime.

In short, since I did not file a police report within 72 hours of the crime, the statute of limitations for reporting the most recent act of sexual assault and molestation as a crime in Florida expired in 1994. I found this extremely narrow window for reporting this crime absurd. I know people who have taken longer to file an insurance claim after a fender bender yet still received full coverage. It was infuriating.

The next action I took was to pursue administrative justice. At around the same time, in the late fall of 2017, I also contacted the Florida Board of Medicine and attempted to file a complaint. In Florida, the Department of Health investigates complaints and reports involving medical doctors who are licensed in the state of Florida.

When necessary, the Department of Health enforces appropriate Florida Statutes. The Department is authorized to take action against health care practitioners in an administrative capacity. These actions may include a reprimand, fine, restriction of practice, remedial education, administrative cost, probation, license suspension, or license revocation. The Department does not, however, represent people who file complaints in civil matters and recommends consulting with a private attorney if that course of action is desired.

I called the Consumer Services office and said that I wanted to file a complaint against a pediatric orthopedist who sexually assaulted and molested me under the guise of medical care in 1990 and 1991. Again, my heart was pounding.

The operator asked me to confirm the dates when these incidents occurred. I told her again, and she quickly informed me that the time limit for filing a complaint had expired. Generally, she said that the statute of limitations is six years from the last date of treatment. Specifically, she told me that for my claim to be considered, I would have needed to file it and have the investigation completed by August 1997, or six years from the date of my last treatment. In 1997, I was finishing graduate school and moving to Chicago for my first job in philanthropy. Any memories of sexual assault and molestation by Dr. Zink were deeply repressed by then.

Before ending the call, the operator informed me that if I was still interested in filing a complaint for an incident that is over six years old, I may do so. However, I would also forfeit my anonymity, according to Florida's rules for reporting complaints to the Board of Medicine, which meant that Dr. Zink would be informed.

I had not been in contact with Zink since being drugged and raped by him in August of 1991and was terrified at the thought that this complaint might result in any form of contact from him. Would he or a member of his office staff call me? I was easy to locate, after all, given my public role as CEO of a community foundation. Would I be sued? I was unfamiliar with the law, and not sure where these types of claims fell. Was he capable of violence and would I or my family be in danger? I wasn't ready to deal with any of this, so I thanked the operator for the information and hung up.

Finally, before the end of 2017, I decided to take action by exploring a path toward civil justice. I contacted a friend, an experienced attorney, for guidance. In doing so, I learned that while the statute of limitations for pursuing civil recourse may offer a course of action given the recent nature of my becoming aware of these repressed memories, typical Florida medical malpractice insurance does not cover such willful acts and the likelihood of recovery of damages would be extremely low. My friend also shared his opinion that a civil trial such as this could be extremely painful for me and my family, given the nature and tactics that Dr. Zink's prior legal counsel had employed in his 1994 trial. He said that it would be likely that my parents, my wife and possibly my children would be deposed, causing undue suffering to them as well as me.

While Stephanie knew about my experience of childhood sexual assault and molestation, I had told neither my parents nor my children about it. I could not imagine what it would be like to have them questioned by an attorney on this subject.

Given this information, what could I do? Gathering more information would be necessary. So, between January 2018 and April 2018, I sought out several people who were involved with the original case against Dr. Zink to learn more from their perspectives:

The columnist who covered Zink's 1994 trial; the district attorney who prosecuted the case; the retired Orlando police detective who led multiple investigations. Each would provide me with helpful insight into the details of the past, along with cold comfort as I recognized the long-lasting damage Zink had done did not start or stop with me alone

16
Looking Back

Betthen January 2018 and April 2018, I spent time trying to gather more information about Dr. Zink's 1994 criminal trial and the circumstances that led up to it. If the current statutes of limitation prevented me from pursuing criminal, administrative, or civil justice, I wanted to have a better understanding of the experiences of the people who were able to take action in the past, albeit unsuccessfully. I made a list of people to contact who I believed could help provide additional background information or insights that could be helpful to me. Some were helpful, and others were dead ends.

One of these people was Debbie Salamone, a former Orlando Sentinel reporter who covered Dr. Zink's 1994 trial. When I reached her by phone, she said she remembered the story even though it had been several years since the trial, during which she had written hundreds of other stories. However, she confirmed that Zink's trial was the only one she had covered related to the specific topic of charges against a doctor of sexual assault and molestation of children. While I was hopeful to find out if anyone else who was not a party to the 1990 or 1994 actions against Dr. Zink had contacted her, she did not have much more helpful information to share. I thanked her for her time, and for the careful reporting she did on this case.

The next person I contacted in my efforts to gain some perspective from those involved with the original case against Dr. Zink was retired Assistant State Attorney and sex crimes prosecutor, Robin Wilkinson. When I called Ms. Wilkinson at her home in April of 2018, I was surprised that she answered. I quickly introduced myself and asked if she would be willing to talk with me. She agreed, and we spent the better part of an hour talking about her experience prosecuting Dr. Zink's past case.

It felt like time travel, with the "adult Jeff" asking questions about a case that could have very well included the "16-year-old Jeff" had

I reported my abuse at the time. Most of my conversation with Ms. Wilkinson consisted of her confirming various elements of the case that were reported publicly. Her voice was flat, matter of fact, but certain in the details.

Before ending the call, I asked her if she believed if the case were tried today, that the outcome might be different?

"I'm not sure," she said. "However, for the sake of those poor boys who I believe told the truth back in 1994 and never got justice, I sure hope so."

I thanked her for her time and for standing up for past victims. It was the least I could do, and enough to motivate me to keep moving forward in my efforts to learn more and pursue justice.

While several of Zink's family members and friends were in attendance at his trial, I could only find public information about his wife and his two children, who were now adults. I wondered if the national news stories and widespread conversations taking place around the MeToo movement prompted Zink's wife to ever revisit the subject of his past criminal charges and trial. Did his children even know?

A Google search resulted in sparse information about Zink's friends who were quoted in the local newspaper, providing words of encouragement and support, at the time of his trial. I was curious to know if any of their opinions about him and his claims that his prior acts were medical had changed?

The last person I contacted in my effort to learn more about the 1994 case against Dr. Zink was Frank Roche. Mr. Roche is the retired Orlando police detective who investigated the case for which Zink was being tried in 1994, and he was also the investigator in the prior case that was dismissed. Finding his contact information took a bit more work.

In August 2013, the Orlando Police published their "Active and Retiree Newsletter" which included pages of photos and comments submitted by current and retired members of the police department and others who care about them. Page 24 of the newsletter included the obituary for retired officer John H. Brewer, who served over 40 years with the Orlando Police Department. In the online comments, Frank Roche wrote the following along with an email address and a phone number:

> *Sorry to hear about the loss of John. We rode together in the early 80s. He had a kind heart. I remember late one night we were taking a break at Dunkin Donuts on S. Orange Ave. when Chief Kolazar walked in to do the same (it was a good laugh at the time). Rest in peace. Thank you, Frank Roche*

I was nervous about calling Frank Roche but hoped that the softer side reflected in his tribute to a fallen colleague was a good sign. I dialed the phone number published in the newsletter, and the person on the other end answered, "Frank Roche," just like every detective show I had ever watched on television.

I introduced myself and told Mr. Roche that I found his name in Orlando Sentinel articles from 1994, indicating that he was the investigating officer in a case against Dr. William Zink. I told him that while I was not a party to that case, I experienced the same as the other victims, and that I would appreciate it if he could answer a few questions for me as I was trying to work through my own experience.

In a polite but firm tone, Roche answered, "I'm sorry, but I'd rather not. That was a long time ago, and I am retired."

I apologized for the interruption and thanked him for his service to the Orlando community.

I was disappointed after hitting another dead end. However, I could empathize with Roche and understand him not wanting to a return to the details of a decades-old case involving the topic of sexual molestation of boys. Veteran cop or not, it would be the last thing that I would want to do if I was in his shoes. Why would anyone want to possibly relive the traumatizing details?

I also imagine that there were specific moments from Roche's career that he had forgotten, and others he had blocked out in order to survive. Moments like the interviews he conducted in the late 80's with the first victims who reported being sexually assaulted and molested by Zink under the guise of medical care. Or moments when perhaps he would stop for a cocktail at an all-night lounge in order to delay returning to his empty house for fear of being alone with the details of the day's investigation. Or moments like when a high-priced defense attorney won a case on a technicality, freeing a serial sex offender with the potential to continue his practice of disguising his abuse as bona fide medical practices.

These memories were a lot for me to even imagine, much less what it must have been like for Roche to live through. I imagine his reply to not get involved was necessary in some capacity in order to be able to live with the idea that, while he did his part, a serial child sex abuser got away with it and was still practicing.

Later, as I reviewed more public information about the case, I was surprised to see how much criticism Detective Roach received from Zink and his legal team for doing what appeared to be textbook investigative work on behalf of child victims of sexual abuse. I was even more surprised to see that Zink and his attorney, Kirkconnell, actually sued the City of Orlando, filing an injunction against Detective Roach in early 1994.

While the records of this case are sealed, the order and descriptions of the various types of judicial proceedings include the appointment of two guardians ad litem. Courts frequently appoint guardians ad litem to represent children's interests in various cases. The guardians ad litem usually act as fact finders for the court, not as advocates for the children.

Given the timing of the court filing and the involvement of guardians ad litem, it is likely that Zink was objecting to a restriction on visitation rights with his own children either while in jail or while out on bail. Was Detective Roach investigating the possibility of Zink abusing his own young daughter and son? Were they being prevented from seeing him for their own good? Given the volume of evidence Roach had uncovered about Zink's behaviors with his young patients, it would not be hard to imagine.

Whatever he was pursuing, I am grateful for Frank Roche's dedication and persistence. Had he not pursued Zink with such dogged determination, I doubt that any of his actions would have come to light. Because of his police work, regardless of whether Zink was convicted or not, I have enough information to know that I am not alone.

What everyone missed, however, was the disturbing patterns that likely began with Zink long before Roche's investigation. Hindsight reveals the tell-tale signs that Zink laid the groundwork for his eventual acts of molestation and sexual assault by grooming his child patients, and in many cases, their parents.

17

Grooming

Looking back, I believe that Dr. Zink groomed me. Why else would I have normalized acts that have repulsed every person I have told since remembering them? Given some of the details of similar behavior by Larry Nasser being reported in the news, I wanted to get a better understanding of this subject.

In my research, I learned that in 1996, a couple of years after Zink's trial, the Clearinghouse on Supervised Visitation was created to provide statewide technical assistance on issues related to the delivery of supervised visitation services in Florida. In 1998, the Clearinghouse published a training manual covering the recommended training content developed by the Florida Supreme Court. In 2004, this content was expanded to produce "Referrals to Supervised Visitation Programs: A Manual for Florida's Judges."

One section of the manual is entitled "The Progression of Sexual Abuse." It could have been called "Grooming." The section includes a description and illustrations that could have been taken directly from the various reports filed by Detective Roach during the years he investigated Zink for crimes of sexual abuse of his pediatric patients.

Although a family member may sexually abuse a child a single time before disclosure, the section reads, the typical pattern of sexual abuse occurs over a period and progresses from normal contact to sexual activity. Sexual abusers often groom a child for abuse, often using secrecy and power and control to get the child to accept increased sexualized contact.

A table in the manual lists the following as examples of the types of acts a perpetrator will move through as he progresses through the cycle of sexual abuse of a child:

- Observing the child bathing, undressing, excreting.
- Nudity on the part of the adult.
- Genital exposure by the adult.

- Kissing, hugging, massaging the child in a lingering inappropriate manner.
- Fondling of the child's breast, buttocks, thighs, genitals.
- Masturbation in presence of the child, or instructing child to masturbate.
- Fellatio or cunnilingus.
- Digital penetration of the vagina, rectum or anus.
- Penile penetration of the vagina, rectum or anus.

Zink was familiar to me, having cared for my younger brother. He went out of his way to show up at the hospital on the evening of my accident. In his office, he watched me undress. He fondled my genitals and digitally penetrated my anus and rectum, first with my father in the exam room and later alone. While I could never see it happening because of the bright light he shined in my face, I suspect that he masturbated while he photographed me in the nude. I know he drugged and raped me – all under the guise of medicine.

I do not ever recall being asked by anyone if anything that Zink did to me made me feel uncomfortable. I certainly was never shown anything that resembled this bulleted list to confirm or deny whether one or more of these acts had taken place with Zink.

Looking at the list now, it is almost like a grooming score board. Zink ran the table. He mastered the game. As a young boy, raised to respect authority and desperate to return to the baseball diamond, I simply thought that is what he was supposed to do.

18
Moving Forward

By May 19, 2018, more than six months had passed since I remembered being sexually assaulted as a child by Dr. William P. Zink for acts that he claimed were medically appropriate. After almost 30 years of denial and repression, spending this time remembering my childhood sexual assault caused feelings of extreme sadness. I grieved for my 16-year-old self who put all of his trust in a doctor in order to heal and return as quickly as possible to the baseball diamond, only to have this trust shattered by repugnant and depraved acts that violate every word of the Hippocratic oath to "first do no harm."

That poor boy.

These memories also caused feelings of extreme rage. I seethed at the thought that while his victims suffered years of adversity, simple searches of Google and Facebook showed that Dr. Zink continued to operate a private practice, maintain an affiliation with AdventHealth Orlando, raise his family, travel, and volunteer all with impunity. I mean, really.

Fuck this guy.

After confirming with the Orlando Police Department, I learned that the only way for my story to make it into the official record, even though the statute of limitations had expired, was to file an official police report. When I called to file the report, the dispatch officer told me that while I could not make my report over the phone, I did not need to come into the police station to file my report. She said that a patrol officer could take my statement from any location in the Orlando area.

While I knew that filing a police report about the details of a decades-old crime would likely have no bearing on Zink's freedom or ability to continue practicing, doing so was important to me. The idea of hearing myself tell my story to a police officer, of seeing the official paperwork that would be filed, felt just as important as my decision to follow my doctor's advice to cope with the acute bouts of anxiety and depression I had been experiencing. It would be more strong medicine to help me heal.

By coincidence, I had a brief trip to Orlando scheduled for the following morning and decided to make my official statement then. On May 19, 2018, I drove from Vero Beach to the Mall at Millenia in Orlando in advance of my brother-in-law's wedding. I needed a new pair of black loafers, and my wife suggested I splurge by trying to find a pair at Farragamo in the Mall at Millenia in Orlando.

I left Vero Beach that morning and made the drive in record time, arriving at a little before 9:30am. The mall opened at 10:00am, so with a half hour to kill, I dialed 9-1-1 to make the police report from my car in the mall parking lot outside Brio Tuscan Grille.

It was surreal, dialing the phone to report a decades-old crime in an empty parking lot from the front seat of my car. No special attention or trauma-informed assistance. Just me, my cup of Starbucks coffee and almost 30 years of pent-up emotions.

After about 90 minutes, a patrol officer named Andrew Merks arrived to take my initial statement. Officer Merks appeared outside of my driver's side window, fresh-faced and rested, as if he had just returned from a vacation. At first, I was concerned that he might think I was wasting his time, reporting crimes that occurred so long ago. His response indicated the exact opposite, taking me seriously from the moment he introduced himself. He was careful, deliberate, asking detailed questions about my experiences that led me to believe that he was already making a case for prosecution in his mind.

"Mr. Pickering, in your own words, please describe what happened to you," Officer Merks began.

I told him about remembering the repressed memories being sexually assaulted and molested as a child by Dr. Zink under the guise of medicine. I explained the details of what happened to me on each of the visits over the roughly 18-month period that he treated me for a knee injury.

"Under Florida statutes, what you are describing can be defined as sexual battery and lewd or lascivious molestation," Merks clarified. "The medical aspect of this may complicate it. Given the number of times you said that the doctor put his finger in your rectum, that sounds unusual. The fondling, that's a different story. Pictures, not sure, but they also sound unusual."

According to Florida statutes, "sexual battery" means oral, anal, or vaginal penetration by, or union with, the sexual organ of another or the anal or vaginal penetration of another by any other object; however, sexual battery does not include an act done for a bona fide medical purpose.

"How old do you estimate the doctor was at the time of the first incident?"

"Probably around 40 years old," I answered. Younger than I was am now. He seemed so much older to me back then. However, he was still a grown man.

"How old were you on the date of the first incident?" Merks asked.

"I was sixteen years old," I answered. Almost the same age as my oldest son, Colin. I remember feeling so mature back then. However, I was still a developing boy.

According to Florida law, a person 18 years of age or older who commits sexual battery upon a person less than 12 years of age commits a capital felony. Capital felonies may carry a sentence of life in prison or death.

As for lewd and lascivious molestation, an offender 18 years of age or older who intentionally touches in a lewd or lascivious manner the breasts, genitals, genital area, or buttocks of a person 16 years of age, but less than 18 years of age, commits a felony of the second degree. Second degree felonies may carry a sentence of prison for up to 15 years.

"Did the doctor restrain you in any way, by force or with a weapon, during the times you saw him," Merks continued. "or did he threaten to do so?"

"No, nothing other than a closed door and turning off the lights," I answered.

According to Florida law, a person who commits sexual battery upon a person 12 years of age or older, without that person's consent, and in the process thereof uses or threatens to use a deadly weapon or uses actual physical force commits a life felony. Life felonies carry a sentence of life in prison. Without threat or force, a person who commits sexual battery upon a person 12 years of age or older, without that person's consent, commits a felony of the first degree. A person convicted of this crime could face a minimum sentence of 30 years in prison.

"Where were your parents during these examinations?" Merks asked.

"Sometimes they were at the doctor's office, but other times I drove myself," I answered.

"Did you ever tell them about these incidents?"

"No," I answered.

Within another 30 minutes, Officer Jaqueline Horner arrived. Officer Horner approached my open driver's side window and introduced herself as a member of the Special Victim Response Team. She was young, possibly in her mid-thirties. Average height and physically fit, with a cross-country runner's build. Even with her bulletproof vest, gun belt and walkie talkie, I do not think she could have weighed more than 130 pounds. Her demeanor was serious and focused.

Officer Horner listened to my story and then asked me to describe my sexual assault and molestation in a sworn written statement. Using my own pen, in cursive handwriting, I wrote the following statement on a carbon form. The white copy would go to the State Attorney, and the yellow copy would go to the Orlando Police Department records.

I became a patient of pediatric orthopedist Dr. William P. Zink, M.D., sometime between 1988 and 1989, seeing him for one or two minor sports injuries during that time, as well as for one or two sports physicals required for school athletics. On February 13, 1990, I was seriously injured while playing catcher in a baseball game at Bishop Moore High School versus Mt. Dora High School. I was transported to Winter Park Memorial Hospital where Dr. Zink visited me in preparation for arthroscopic surgery on my left knee the following day. On February 14, 1990, Dr. Zink performed surgery, visited me in the recovery room and scheduled a follow-up appointment to be held in his office at 61 West Columbia Street, Orlando, within the week. At the follow-up appointment, Dr. Zink evaluated the cast on my left leg and recommended it be recast. Before leaving the appointment, Dr. Zink performed an ungloved rectal examination and examined my genitals. Following the appointment and through September of 1991 when I left for college, I visited Dr. Zink's office for numerous follow-up appointments to monitor the healing of my knee, the progress of my physical therapy, the fit of various knee braces, and for regular sports physicals. At each appointment, ungloved rectal exams and genital exams were performed. On several occasions, without a parent present, I was taken into a room in a back office for a procedure Dr. Zink called a "moire." Dr. Zink turned on an overhead light, turned on a spotlight, required me to undress and lower my underwear while he took photos. Florida Hospital website lists his current office at 2909 N. Orange Avenue, Suite 102. To my recollection, these actions were committed without a threat of violence to me or my family, or without restraint. I may have been taking pain medication, but not under influence of sedative or anesthesia other than the surgery. It was my impression that all of these procedures were required for my treatment. However, had I known these acts were of a sexual nature I would not have consented. I am reporting this crime after recent media stories of sexual assault in similar circumstances that caused me to recall my own experience. I am in town for other personal reasons and took the opportunity to file the report while in Orlando. My participation in these acts was based on my understanding that these procedures were required in order to be cleared to participate in future athletic activities. Until a recent conversation with my wife and psychologist, I have never reported this crime. If the statute of limitations has not expired, I wish to press charges and testify. I recall these acts occurred at least 12 times.

After reading my written statement, Officer Horner used the laptop computer in her patrol car to confirm that Dr. Zink had 10 closed cases in Orange County Court system for sexual battery and other sexual crimes against children where he was found not guilty. She told me that the office where my crimes took place at 61 Columbia Street no longer existed, but that Dr. Zink was now practicing as an orthopedic surgeon at 2909 N. Orange Avenue, Suite 102, Orlando, Florida and was affiliated with AdventHealth Orlando. She informed me that while I was interested in pressing charges, the statute of limitations had expired. Several factors contributed to this including the fact that I was 16 at the time of the crime (and not younger), as well as the fact that no police report was filed within 72 hours of the incident.

"What happens next?" I asked.

Officer Horner told me that my report would be used for documentation purposes. If any new reports are filed, it could be used for context or other witness testimony.

Officer Horner ended our time by notifying her supervisors, and by providing me with a Sexual Violence Pamphlet and a Victims Rights Booklet. Two shitty pieces of paper, likely printed in the office.

I felt confused. I felt dissatisfied. I felt relieved. My secret was out. I also felt anxious, not knowing what might come of this. Considering how serious the police officers were with their detailed questions, I felt some comfort. They believed me.

For the first time, I realized that there was real value in speaking up and giving a statement. For the first time, I experienced the importance of being heard by a stranger and being believed. In my case, the stranger happened to be two sworn law enforcement officers, and my experience gave me an honest glimpse into at least one part of the criminal justice system that is good because of the integrity and sound training of its people.

I texted Stephanie and told her that I did it. I felt proud of myself, that I deserved something special.

Like a new pair of shoes. Black leather slip-on loafers.

The Ferragamos were too narrow. Gucci fit just right.

19
Tell Me More

On September 7, 2018, after confirming that Dr. William P. Zink was still practicing medicine and affiliated with AdventHealth, I mailed letters to Daryl Tol, President and CEO of Advent-Health Central Florida and Dr. David Moorhead, Chief Medical Officer at Florida Hospital AdventHealth. My letters detailed my experience of childhood sexual assault under the guise of medical care by Dr. William P. Zink, informed them of his continued affiliation with AdventHealth and requested their assistance in pursuing a remedy that might prevent similar acts in the future.

Several weeks later, I received a phone call from Melissa Dobias, Executive Director of Risk Management, following up on my letter. She acknowledged receipt of my letter and explained that the details had been reviewed. She said that while she was sorry to hear about my experience, at the time of my surgery, Winter Park Memorial Hospital was not yet affiliated with AdventHealth. The acquisition of 50-plus-year-old community hospital was completed in 2000.

I told Dobias that while I was not familiar with the law related to such transactions, I was certain that the public perception of Winter Park residents was that damaged goods or not, AdventHealth owned the house, ghosts and all. Winter Park is a small town. Surely there must be some practice for at least looking into incidents like the one I was reporting. Unfortunately, she said, there was not.

I told her that from my review of AdventHealth's website, it appeared that Dr. Zink was employed by the organization. Technically, she explained that he was not an employee but rather a member of the medical staff. Did that mean he still had privileges to perform surgery in one or more of the Advent Hospitals? Yes, it did, she answered. Then given what had been publicly reported years ago, and what I was reporting now, was there any way for me to get AdventHealth to revoke his privileges or join a complaint against his medical license. Unfortunately, she replied, neither was possible as it is a complicated matter.

I was frustrated, angry, and felt betrayed. I was a Winter Park native. My younger brothers were both born at Winter Park Memorial Hospital. My mother worked in the hospital's intensive care unit as a nurse for 30 years until she retired. Many of the doctors whom I had looked up to as a child as role models and who inspired my early interest in medicine spent their careers caring for patients within those hospital walls. Several remained on the hospital's board of trustees. But it did not count for anything. It was a complicated matter.

Then, I received a written response dated October 17, 2018, which read:

> *Dear Mr. Pickering,*
>
> *I would like to thank you again for taking time to speak with me about the concerns you outlined in the letter you sent to Dr. David Moorhead on September 7, 2018. We do take this seriously and we take steps to ensure the safety of our patients as a standard practice. While we have sympathy for your circumstance, the situation you described did not occur at Florida Hospital and we are unable to join you in your request to take action against Dr. Zink's medical license. If you have anything else you wish to discuss, please contact me at 407.200.1322.*
>
> *Respectfully,*
> *Mellissa Dobias*
> *Executive Director, Risk Management*

I was disappointed, but not necessarily surprised by this response.

I called Ms. Dobias at the number she provided and asked her if she could provide me with an explanation for the business reasons the AdventHealth system and Florida Hospital would maintain an affiliation with someone of Dr. Zink's reputation. She could not.

I also asked her if she could explain how maintaining an affiliation with someone of Dr. Zink's reputation aligned with the organization's expressly stated charitable mission of "Extending the Healing Ministry of Christ." She could not.

For months, I wondered if any change would result from my efforts to bring this to the attention of the AdventHealth leadership team. Perhaps there were legal or other contractual reasons why the organization could not take action against Dr. Zink. However, word of my inquiry could have been passed along. After years of operating in the clear, maybe Zink would feel the heat and decide to move on or retire.

Periodic checks of the AdventHealth website, however, indicated otherwise. Zink was still practicing as a member of the organization's medical staff.

More than a year after my letters to Darryl Tol and David Moorhead, in January 2020, I posed the same questions to AdventHealth CEO, Terry Shaw, in an online message through LinkedIn. Given all the information that has been shared publicly about Dr. Zink, I was interested in talking with Mr. Shaw to understand his business purpose for maintaining an affiliation with Dr. Zink.

I shared my personal mobile phone number and invited a conversation about my experience. I did not threaten legal action, and I did not demand financial compensation. I simply asked him for his ear.

Knowing that Mr. Shaw is a busy man, I did not expect to hear back right away, but I did follow up weekly with a reminder of my interest in talking. I waited patiently for his reply.

I never heard back from Terry Shaw.

I did read news, however, of AdventHealth's recent launch of its Innovation Lab, sort of a "think and do" space for physicians, researchers and other professionals to develop their ideas for medical devices and other interventions. This was a bold initiative that Mr. Shaw cited as an example of the organization's commitment to patient-centered care. Given this development, I thought that Shaw might have a more empathetic response to the one that I had previously received from his colleagues. That would not be the case.

As a graduate of Stanford University's Hasso Plattner School of Design, otherwise known as the "d.school," and former student of IDEO and d.school founder, David Kelly, I know that there are three words that inform the work of places like AdventHealth's Innovation Lab. They are "tell me more."

"Tell me more" is what human-centered design relies on in order to uncover the intimate details about a patient's positive or negative experience with a doctor affiliated with your hospital or health care system.

"Tell me more" is what invites patients to lean in and whisper the painful or embarrassing details of something that a doctor affiliated with your hospital or health care system did to them under the guise of medical care.

"Tell me more" gets the hard-to-hear answer that a doctor who is still affiliated with your health care system, when treating me for a knee injury, put his ungloved finger in my rectum, fondled my genitals, and took nude photos of me without a parent present on multiple occasions over a period of 18 months when I was a child.

"Tell me more" is what gives a grown man like me the belief that it is worth it to share the uncomfortable experience of telling my story to the chief executive officer of one of the most respected hospital systems in the United States, if it can result in a business decision to discontinue a relationship with a serial child sex abuser.

No one in a leadership role at AdventHealth was giving me or the community the courtesy of an explanation as to how the decision to remain affiliated with Dr. William P. Zink makes business sense or how it demonstrates the organization's mission of "Extending the Healing Ministry of Christ."

I desperately wanted to hear Terry Shaw say, "Tell me more." All I heard was deafening silence.

20

With Time Ticking, Finding My Superpower

With statutes of limitation preventing criminal and administrative action, my final path forward toward justice began in November 2018, as I explored the possibility of pursuing civil action against Zink. To build a case and ultimately file a civil claim, I would need to hire an experienced attorney to help guide me through the legal process. Before doing so, however, I was curious to know more about the requirements of filing a civil lawsuit in the state of Florida. I was also curious to know if there were any assets worth pursuing. While money was not my primary motivation, I knew that it could be a meaningful way to punish someone like Zink.

I had spent the better part of my entire professional career working as a philanthropic advisor with high-net-worth individuals and families. I was highly skilled at using publicly available information in order to identify and qualify prospective clients with whom I ultimately wanted to pursue doing business. It was a method that I had used for almost 25 years to raise hundreds of millions of dollars for the greater good, and now it was a "superpower" that I would use to fight back against Zink and the system that has allowed him to avoid prison and remain in practice.

Unlike the criminal law process, which punishes abusers if they are found guilty beyond a reasonable doubt, civil lawsuits compensate survivors of sexual abuse when they are able to show that it is more likely than not that the defendant committed the act. I wondered what was required in order to file a civil lawsuit against Zink, and what it ultimately would take to win.

Fortunately, there were numerous resources available online that detailed the requirements for filing a civil suit in Florida and the various legal theories that may be employed. I would need to prove a cause of action by Zink that involved assault, battery, intentional infliction of emotional distress or negligent infliction of emotional distress.

Surprisingly, my age at the time of Zink's first act of sexual assault and molestation – 16 – made a significant difference on the statute of limitations for filing a claim. Had I been younger, no statute of limitations existed. In my case, however, a complex formula pertained, given that I did not remember the assault until nearly 30 years later. Time was ticking.

Equally surprising, Zink's insistence that his actions were medical in nature would also play a role if I were to pursue civil action. While unlikely to be permitted in today's medical protocol or condoned in current culture, Zink's claims that rectal examinations and nude photographs of boys were for bona fide medical purposes had some influence on the outcome of his prior criminal trial. This would likely be factored into a judge or jury's consideration of a civil claim.

With a few clicks of a mouse, it was very easy for me to pull together information and come up with an estimate of Zink's net worth and determine whether he possessed resources that could be used to pay a judgement against him. I learned that Zink had assets, but like many wealthy individuals, he was using clever legal and accounting structures in order to shield them from liability. Just knowing this, however, gave me the energy I needed to keep digging and gathering more information that I could use to my advantage.

According to information listed on the Florida Division of Corporation's website, "Fausse Rivere" is the name of the limited liability corporation that holds the Orlando, Florida, home and assets of Dr. William P. Zink. These two French words nearly jumped off the computer screen as I skimmed the alphabetized listings under the letter "Z."

"Fausse Rivere," a horse-shoe lake in Pointe Coupee, Louisiana, was once part of the Mississippi River until it changed course in 1722, leaving a lake that the French named. In English it means "False River," and is the eponymous title of the latest album by my friend, New Orleans songsmith and troubadour, Andrew Duhon. His songs from this record and the previous Grammy-nominated The Moorings had been an intimate part of my healing journey since the fall of 2017.

After finding "Fausse Rivere" on the Florida Division of Corporation's website, I also learned that Zink is the registered agent for two more LLCs named "JRZ Investments" and "NLZ Investments." JRZ likely stood for the initials of Zink's adult son, and NLZ likely stood for the initials of his adult daughter. Publicly available photos on social media of family celebrations and vacations suggest privilege and the benefits that come with it.

Once I finally decided to pursue civil action, I hired an attorney who assisted me in drafting a demand letter, which I eventually mailed to Zink and his associates including the insurance company that issues his medical malpractice insurance. Their reply was to claim no liability for his willful acts of sexual battery or molestation. No coverage, therefore, no resources to pay attorneys' fees and damages. Their reply went on to claim that Dr. Zink himself has no personal resources that can be used to compensate victims.

Bullshit.

Assuming Zink has at least earned the average annual starting salary of $350,000 for a Florida pediatric orthopedist, over 30 years this would put Dr. Zink's earnings at $10 million. Given the highly specialized services of a pediatric orthopedist, combined with the demands of major metropolitan community with a thriving youth sports culture, it is likely that Zink's career earnings were well beyond $10 million given his veteran status.

Other than the public report of two settlements with anonymous minor plaintiffs in 1990 and 1992, both of which were procured by Orlando attorney Keith Mitnick, no other restitution has been paid.

Instead, it is millions for Zink, his family, and the businesses he associated with, and not one cent for his victims. If that is not a false river, I do not know what is.

21

Finding My Own Voice, With a Little Help from My Friends

As 2020 approached, I made the difficult but necessary decision to go public with my story. Although there was a seemingly endless string of stories of similar childhood sexual assault and molestation being covered in the news media at the time, none of them were like mine. After running into so many dead ends, I believed going public could help me and that it might help others.

Taking action and making decisions like this is part of my nature. I like to get things done, for myself and for other people.

In baseball as a child, when a runner on the opposing team took his lead from first base and threatened to steal, I wanted him to break for second in order to have the chance to throw him out. If bases were loaded and a passed ball meant losing the game, I was the half of the battery who was unafraid to call for a hard-breaking curve ball, knowing that I could block any pitch that happened to skid in the dirt as the batter swatted an off-balance swing to strike out and end the inning.

Because getting on base mattered most to my team's ability to score runs and win, I was the right-handed batter who was tough enough to crowd the plate and get hit by a pitch thrown too far inside . . . off my left shoulder blade, my rib cage, my left elbow, my butt, my thigh, the outside of my left knee, my left ankle, the top of my back right foot. I was playing Moneyball before Moneyball was a thing.

For the past two years, I had already been making strides, getting on base. It was starting to feel as if the bases were loaded. Time to swing for the fences.

On January 20, 2020, when I contacted AdventHealth CEO Terry Shaw online through LinkedIn, I told him that February would mark 30 years since I was sexually assaulted and molested by a pediatric orthopedic surgeon over a period of 18 months under the guise of medical care. I informed him that this doctor remained affiliated with AdventHealth. Although the firm's risk manager wrote to me the year before claiming no ability to help, I respectfully asked him to reconsider. I included my personal mobile phone number and invited him to call.

After a week passed without hearing from Shaw, I sent another message through LinkedIn still offering the opportunity to talk about my experience and the ongoing affiliation of my abuser with AdventHealth. I appreciated his busy schedule and encouraged him to contact me at his convenience.

Crickets. I could not believe it that a fellow CEO who was provided the professional courtesy of a private opportunity to discuss such a troubling matter would not take me seriously by making a simple phone call.

My first instinct was to contact a reporter in the Orlando media market who might be sympathetic to my story. Before doing so, I sought counsel from a childhood friend, Kari, who had a long, distinguished career as a television news producer.

After listening to my story and telling me how sorry she was to learn about what happened to me, Kari asked me if I wanted to know her point of view about how to proceed. She did not offer unsolicited advice. Instead, she asked me for permission to share her wisdom. What she said changed the course of my journey.

To offer some perspective, Kari shared the intimate details of two stories that she had been assigned to pursue related to similar accounts of sexual abuse and molestation of child and young adult athletes. The professional journalists on her team were responsible for documenting the facts, and for uncovering leads that might shed more light on the story's subjects. Some of their work involved getting close to victims, listening to the details of their experiences, and then framing what they learned in a format that could be consumed by millions of readers and viewers.

While Kari and her team maintained the highest level of journalistic integrity in the process of getting close to victims, she suggested that the instant these stories were published, they would be "owned" by someone else. How the victims would be portrayed and how their stories would be interpreted would be up to someone else. The story would no longer be theirs.'

Up to someone else to accept or dismiss. Up to someone else to believe or to judge. Up to someone else to empathize with or to criticize. Up to someone else to rally behind or to shy away from.

In sharing their story, these victims and survivors lost more control than they gained. They lost ownership of their stories. In some ways, they also lost an authentic voice.

I didn't want to be in a situation where my story was no longer my own, so I decided that I would keep my story to myself until I was ready to tell it. When I was ready to tell it, I would tell it in my own words, using my own method, through my own channel. It would be my truth, and it would set me free.

With a little help from my friends, I began to find my own voice.

22
Hearing My Own Voice,
With a Little Help from My Friends

My next step was inspired by Terry Gross, host of the radio program Fresh Air which is broadcast from WHYY in Philadelphia and distributed by National Public Radio. For more than 40 years, Gross has interviewed a roster of guests whose art, inventions, publications, and otherwise meaningful work interest her and the five million listeners who regularly tune in. I was one of those long-time listeners.

Terry Gross' style is at the same time comforting while curious, inspiring while inquisitive, sensitive while straightforward, thoughtful while thought-provoking. Even if it was in private, I wanted to tell my story to someone like her, who could help me get it out and then give me something to listen to and reflect on as a totem against which to mark my progress.

My friend Tania, who works as a journalist, graphic designer, photographer, and vocalist, offered to help. I first met her while working together on the estate of a client who had recently passed away after complications from throat cancer. Without family or heirs, before his death, he entrusted Tania with the responsibility of distributing his assets to friends and the charitable causes he loved, which included my foundation and the local opera. I have always believed this to be sacred work and was impressed by Tania's reverence of the task at hand. I believed she would demonstrate the same care and concern with my story.

I asked Tania to meet for coffee to discuss a personal project that I wanted to know if she could help with. We met on the patio of an ice cream and coffee shop across the street from a beachside park where children played on new equipment that our foundation had helped to pay for. I was not nervous or ashamed about what I was prepared to tell her. I had listened to many of Tania's radio stories and knew that she would be a good listener. I gave a tearful, first-hand account of my story, and it moved her. We were relatively new friends, yet I felt her empathy.

Tania asked for a week or so to think about the best way to approach my interview. I was grateful when she called and told me her extremely thoughtful idea. Tania understood my intention that the interview be recorded for my own use and not for public distribution. However, she approached the process with the same level of professionalism she would for any other interview subject.

Instead of scheduling my interview in a recording studio or some other formal location, Tania suggested she simply come to my home and talk with Stephanie and me as we made dinner. The kids had been asking me to make a special dish of shrimp and swordfish curry, so we set a date for an upcoming Sunday evening.

When Tania arrived, I opened the west-facing front door to our home to see her smiling face and outstretched arms backlit by the setting sun, offering a bottle of wine and a hug to both Stephanie and me. I told her the kids were down on the beach, so we had about an hour to prepare dinner and talk before getting invaded.

Tania quickly arranged a simple microphone and recording device on the counter that separated our kitchen from our dining room. It was close enough to the area where I was preparing dinner. Tania pulled up a bar stool as Stephanie poured the wine.

I introduced myself as I started by chopping and sautéing the peppers and onions that, when combined with fish stock and curry spices, made a roux that would simmer for 15 minutes. Stephanie did the same.

"Last time we talked, you and I discussed the recent news of sexual abuse of nearly 500 young athletes over the course of two decades by predatory trainer Dr. Larry Nasser," Tania continued. "Many have since wondered how did he get away with it? And for so long? You have your own experience to share that might shed some light on those questions."

I began telling Tania about how I was abused by my own sports doctor over the course of 18 months, starting when I was 16. "It was 30 years ago," I told her. "And I recently discovered this doctor is still licensed and practicing."

I measured out two cups of basmati rice, rinsed it, and poured it in the rice steamer along with a tablespoon of coconut oil and a quarter teaspoon of Madagascar vanilla extract. While the recipe did not call for it, I liked the way the subtle hint of tropical flavor, when combined with the seafood and curry, transported me across the globe to a jungle-side beach somewhere in the Bay of Bengal.

"After doing some research of my own, I soon discovered that the laws currently in place make it impossible for me to stop this doctor from practicing and potentially abusing others. Too much time has passed, according to Florida's statutes of limitations."

"How long did it take for you to remember?" Tania asked. "Did you tell anyone?"

I told Tania that I kept this secret for 30 years. "I actually did not even remember the numerous accounts of being sexually assaulted and molested until the fall of 2017. I remembered during a conversation with Stephanie, and that changed everything. It was the start of many more conversations about this terrible memory."

While the recipe called for one pound of shrimp, I peeled and deveined two pounds and dropped them into the cast-iron pot. With three hungry kids returning shortly from their ocean swim, I figured I could always refrigerate leftovers. With my sharpest paring knife, I removed the skin and the bloodline from three swordfish filets. I cut them in half and laid them on top of the shrimp and the simmering roux.

"What you describe happening to you sounds awful," Tania remarked. "Is it common for victims to not remember these experiences, or to keep them secret for so long?"

I told Tania about what I had learned from a number of organizations with resources to help people like me who have experienced sexual assault and molestation. RAINN's National Sexual Assault Hotline at 1-800-656-HOPE was one of the first places I called to find information and resources. The nonprofit charitable organization 1in6.org helped me to understand the unique experiences of male survivors of sexual assault. ChildUSA, the think-tank for child protection, was extremely helpful for understanding the complications associated with sex abuse crimes and related statutes of limitations. "Statistics show that most victims of childhood sexual abuse sometimes do not fully remember or reveal it for decades. It can be even harder for males to speak about their experiences."

"Take me back to the time of your injury," Tania suggested. "What happened?"

I told Tania about growing up in Winter Park, about my family and about playing baseball throughout my childhood and into high school. I told her about the game where I was injured, about my trip to the hospital and the surgery, and about the abuse that began at the start of my recovery and lasted until I went away to college.

"From the very beginning, this doctor's behavior was very similar to that of Larry Nassar," Stephanie offered. "He had endeared himself to Jeff's parents, and then Jeff – his victim – had to continue to come back because he promised them that he'd get him better."

To finish the dish, the recipe called for the zest and juice of one lime to be added for the last two minutes of cooking. Earlier in the day, I had stopped by my friend's house for a special ingredient. She and her husbandlive down the road in the island neighborhood here called Riomar. Their family had been in the citrus business in Florida for decades, and he had a grove of specialty fruit trees behind his house that included a Kaffir lime tree. I found its juice and zest to be the perfect combination of sweet and sour, pairing perfectly with the curry dish. It also made for a better gin and tonic.

I continued by telling Tania about the numerous visits I made to Dr. Zink's office over the course of 18 months, and about what he did to me on each of those visits. I told her about the strange photographs he took of me, about the dark room cluttered with photos of other boys, about how he instructed me to pull down my underwear. I told her about everything, how embarrassing it was, and how I didn't tell anyone.

"I was embarrassed, ashamed, freaked out. From then on, I was always worried that I was going to have that done again."

I told her about the panic attacks, the phantom pain I had experienced right before leaving for college. The relief I needed, the agony I endured, and how it all ended.

"Then I buried it, and from that point on I never went back. I never saw the guy again or ever mentioned it to anybody until I told Stephanie."

We sat for a moment, listening to the sound of the waves and the chatter of children coming in from the beach.

Stephanie added, "Jeff and I discovered that a few years after he stopped seeing this doctor, while Jeff was away at college, this doctor was charged criminally for similar acts committed against other patients. Multiple boys had come forward accusing him of the same abuse."

"Ultimately he was acquitted," I told Tania. "His defense was that there was 'a misunderstanding between the science and the art of medicine.' And to this day, I think the doctor stands behind that and believes that what he did was medically appropriate."

I plated the shrimp and swordfish curry and handed a dish to each of the kids as they filed through the kitchen. Stephanie transferred the naan that was warming in the oven to the table. I said a blessing.

We agreed to continue the conversation after dinner. Tania wanted to talk particularly about what has helped me to cope with the difficulties brought on by remembering these traumatic experiences. I made a mental note to tell her how important it was for me to eventually ask for help, to seek professional assistance, to share my story with a few good friends whom I knew I could trust and who would make me feel safe. I wanted to tell her how important it was that I was believed from the start.

By this point in my healing journey, the family members, friends and professionals with whom I chose to share my story all responded by saying words like "I believe you" and "I'm so sorry this happened to you" and "I am here for you."

These close, confidential, incredibly emotional disclosures were met with replies that helped me to stop being so afraid of what had happened to me and of what I had been unable to remember or share for so long. I heard statements such as "You can tell me as much, or as little as you want." I heard the words "It is not your fault." I felt relief when someone said "I'm glad you told me" and "I'm so proud of you."

Nobody asked, "Why?"

As it turns out, there is an entire global movement and campaign called "Start by Believing." It is an effort that was started by End Violence Against Women International, and it is focused on transforming the way our global society and our individual communities respond to sexual assault. The movement's website, www.startbybelieving.org, includes several extremely helpful resources to help guide individuals, corporations, and communities in their efforts to be better listeners, better supporters, and better advocates for victims of sexual assault.

For now, however, we would enjoy a family dinner together and show gratitude for the fresh air brought into our home by a special guest.

When Tania finally finished editing our interview, hearing my own voice tell my story of childhood sexual abuse was both sad and comforting.

Sad because it made a tragic story true. The unwavering voice that I had only previously heard play back in my head, now reverberated in my own ears, making it so.

Comforting because it provided hard evidence of someone believing me. Stephanie's first-hand account of being the first to hear my story, followed by Tania's gentle coaxing of the details, gave me hope.

I heard my own voice, with a little help from my friends.

23
Writing in My Own Voice, With a Little Help from My Friends

As an introvert and someone who has fully embraced my Generation X traits, other than team sports or professional associations, I have never been a joiner. Crowds exhaust me, and while my career and certain artistic pursuits have put me in situations where I am the center of attention, I much prefer privacy and the stakes that come with relying on myself.

My tendencies toward self-reliance and independence have always been fostered by my ability to generate my own motivation rather than rely on the encouragement of others. I generally decline offers of help, and usually remain demure when complimented.

After listening to the recording of my story that Tania made for me, Stephanie told me how proud she was of me. Both she and Tania encouraged me to do more, perhaps write an article or an essay about my experience. Put more of this out into the world.

The idea of writing my story terrified me in the same way that getting bumped by a shark did years before on a surf trip to Santa Cruz. Cold, steel gray water and sky. White death lurking just below the surface, and the only way out, to survive, was to paddle and ride the wave.

For inspiration, I drew from my longstanding admiration of an extended family member and friend, Dan Sinker. Since meeting Dan in Chicago in the early Nineties, I had been inspired by the do-it-yourself spirit that seemed to infuse every project he made come to life. Dan's "We Owe You Nothing," a collection of interviews with some of punk rock's pioneers, torchbearers, and prophets, with their fierce independence and maker mentalities, is electricity in print. The jolt I got from reading it for the first time, the pangs of creative hunger, was the source I tapped when putting pen to paper to write the first words of a serial blog I called "Still Practicing? #MeToo." If conformity and deference to authority got me into this mess, I decided that a little bit of punk rock sensibility would be needed to get me out.

I decided I would write 18 chapters of the blog, one for each of the months that I was sexually assaulted and molested by Dr. Zink. I chose February 14, 2020, as the day I would release the first chapter on social media – 30 years since the fateful day that a knee injury and surgery would forever link me to Zink. With the click of a mouse to post the following words, my story was live and available for the world to sign up and follow along.

Okay, friends. Here goes. After 30 years of silence, the last two of which have included suffering, healing, and pursuing justice, I am joining the growing cloud of witnesses who have had the courage to say #MeToo and #TimesUp by sharing my story. If you would like to receive a daily email of the prologue and subsequent chapters over the next 18 days, you may do so by clicking the link below and providing your email address. I am doing this with hopes of helping others and raising awareness for efforts by organizations like CHILD USA to change statutes of limitations (SOLs) that prevent victims across the nation from pursuing justice.

At first, a handful of close friends and family members entered their email addresses. A contract of sorts, inviting the subsequent chapters of my story to make its way into their inboxes so they could follow me on this journey. Then it was dozens, then hundreds. Dear friends, family members, childhood acquaintances, new colleagues, strangers, all reading along together. I was nerve-wracked about what I had just put into the world, but the kindness of this newly assembled cloud of witnesses to my vulnerability and truth quickly changed that.

What was I so afraid of? I imagined a "big bang" of sorts, with the fragments of my story of childhood sexual abuse being scattered across a modern universe. Zeros and ones, bits and bytes, unstable radioactive particles, nestling into every crack and corner of my universe. Their cancerous half-lives would outlast Zink and me, and eventually decay into infinity.

What resulted, however, was more like nuclear fusion, generating the same energy that powers our sun and the stars. A kind social media post combined with a thoughtful text, bathed me in the light and warmth of a morning sunrise cast on a canyon floor. A soothing voicemail followed by a carefully worded email submerged me in the roiling boil of a post-surf hydrothermal soak. A gentle hug from my daughter followed by a kiss on the cheek from my oldest son draped me in the billowy cover of my favorite down blanket.

Writing and sending my story out was a meditation for me. Assigning words to what had otherwise been wordless up until this point in my life just helped. It helped.

Everything I wrote became a supernova. Scrawled words that mattered most to me and generated their own radiant energy.

I wrote my own voice, with a little help from my friends.

24

Sharing My Own Voice, With a Little Help from My Friends

Writing my story in a daily blog post was helping me to heal. I soon learned that sharing it helped others to heal, too.

In typical do-it-yourself fashion, I had learned how to use various online communications tools to get my story to as many people as I could. Rather than impose on family and friends, my first post to my Facebook account invited anyone who was interested in reading my story to sign up for a daily email that I would distribute using MailChimp. One of the functions built into this online tool is the ability to see who was opening and reading each email, and who was clicking through to a website I created to learn more. Seeing this list of active readers grow to more than 500 people in a matter of days was empowering. Receiving emails of encouragement from friends and strangers was also helping my confidence to grow.

One of the people who was following my daily blog posts was Richard Beene. While I first met Richard in 2010 as president and chief executive officer of The Bakersfield Californian, I didn't really get to know him until a sweltering July evening the following summer when he hosted a house concert featuring Tennessee singer-songwriter Jill Andrews performing original alt-country ballads to a crowd more accustomed to the likes of Buck Owens and Merle Haggard. Our mutual appreciation for the Americana sound eventually evolved into a joint venture we founded with several other friends called "Passing Through Productions."

Our passion for great music brought the finest up and coming roots-rocking solo singer-songwriters, duos and bands to Bakersfield, California as they were traveling between Los Angeles, San Francisco, and Las Vegas. In exchange these troubadours got to eat, sleep and drink well, while making a little extra traveling money by performing for the most appreciative audience in the country. Roots, rock, a respite from the road, and a promise that they would be passing through again.

In retirement, Beene hosted a daily radio show produced by American General Media and KERN, where he applied his veteran journalistic perspective to issues that mattered to residents of Bakersfield, California, and California's southern San Joaquin Valley.

One of the topics he had been covering was the fallout and ongoing controversy surrounding the Diocese of Fresno's recent suspension of Monsignor Craig Harrison, a beloved pastor of St. Francis Parish in Bakersfield. The Diocese's decision was influenced, in part, by the findings of a lengthy investigation by the Fresno County District Attorney's office that found credible reason that Monsignor Harrison had engaged in sexually inappropriate behavior with a young man from another parish in the 1990s. While no charges were filed due to California's statute of limitations at the time, the news was tearing the closely-knit farming and oil town apart.

Beene knew how much I loved the Bakersfield community and the many friends my family made during our time there. It is where Stephanie and I bought our first home as a married couple, where she adopted Colin and Olivia, and where Grant was eventually born. He also knew that I had attended St. Francis Parish, and that my children attended St. Francis Parish School.

When Beene called to invite me to be a guest on his radio show, he did not need to mention the connection between my experience and the tragic events playing out among Bakersfield's faithful. As a former member of the Bakersfield business community, the fact that a high-profile local leader like me had gone public with an account of childhood sexual abuse was newsworthy enough.

As a friend, however, Richard was careful and thoughtful enough to offer his show as an opportunity for me to tell my story. We both agreed that my story would give his listeners a chance to hear a separate but related experience to the one that was being discussed at every lunch table at Luigi's, over Picon punch and plates of pickled tongue at Woolgrower's, and many places in between.

We scheduled my interview for February 26, 2020. A few minutes before 4pm East Coast Time, I got situated at my desk and dialed the station number that Richard provided me to call in as a live, on-air guest. Richard's engineer answered, and after exchanging a few quick words about the Bakersfield weather, the price of oil and the gypsy jazz guitarist, Frank Vignola, performing that night at Buck Owens' Crystal Palace, he put me in the queue to wait for my introduction.

Despite being an experienced public speaker, I was nervous. In the past, while living in Bakersfield, I had been on Richard's show several times, either promoting local philanthropy or an upcoming house concert. Other than the private conversations with family and friends, however, I had never spoken publicly about my experience as a survivor of sexual assault. That was about to change with a twang and a drawl as Richard's voice made its way across the country more than 3,000 miles into my headset.

Instead of listening to Richard's intro live, I muted my microphone, closed my eyes, and listened to the seven-second delay being broadcast over the air. At this moment, I didn't need to be the radio-show guest. Instead, I needed to be the all-American boy with my favorite toy the Ravyns sang about in their 1984 hit "Raised on the Radio."

"When I see sunshine out there and a beautiful day, I think of the people who brighten my life. One of them happens to be on the phone, from Vero Beach, Florida, Mr. Jeff Pickering. He's the former head of our Kern Community Foundation. Mr. Pickering was here for five years, or something like that, and is now the CEO of the Indian River Community Foundation.

Jeff's story is an important one, and I'm going to let him tell it. He's going to explain what happened to him when he was a child, a boy of just 16 years old, who was injured in a baseball game and went to the family doctor and was subjected to multiple occasions of abuse.

He's going to talk about why it took him three decades to come forward. Three decades to deal with guilt and the shame and the embarrassment of it. Three decades to share the story with his wife.

Jeff's story speaks to the abuse that goes on in this country, and why it is important to listen to the accusers. You don't have to believe them 100 percent of the time, but you damn well better not dismiss them with such a cavalier attitude.

People are in pain here. We don't know what people have been through. Jeff Pickering, welcome to the program."

There was something so intimate, so comforting, about the low hum and drawl of Richard's intro to the broadcast coming into my ears. It was not the anonymous tone of mission control. It was not the static dispatch of an astronaut calling in from outer space. It was the plastic silver 9-volt radio heart that Dave Alvin crooned about so many years ago clicking on, music starting, calming my nerves. Just like that, I was talking with an old friend.

I began by telling Richard that while I wished the topic was something more enjoyable, I believed that it was important to talk about. I appreciated his invitation to come on his show.

"Let's get right to it. I count myself fortunate enough to call you a friend. To say that we were shocked about what you wrote is an understatement. You've been publishing a serial blog online, which is now 15 chapters, is going to go 18. I have read them all. Absolutely gripping, terrifying, heartbreaking. It hits all my emotions. You go back and remember exactly what happened to you, and you take us through. Let me ask you, what was it that triggered the thought that I need to deal with this?"

I told Richard and his listeners about the conversation I had with Stephanie in the Fall of 2017, the memories that were triggered by the various #MeToo stories being reported in the news, our online research and discovery that the doctor who sexually assaulted and molested me as a child under the guise of medicine was still practicing, the panic, the depression, and finally the decision to do something about it. I talked about the two-plus years I had spent trying to heal and to pursue justice at the same time. I told him about the healing and justice I hoped would result, and also about the healing and justice that would never happen.

"Do you know when you look back on it why you kept it in? Why you didn't tell someone? I mean, you didn't even tell your wife."

I explained that I didn't think I even remember the sexual assault and molestation, and that I believed it was a repressed memory that did not get shaken loose until it was safe for my brain to do so. When I did remember, my memory was crystal clear. I remembered every detail of what had happened to me, and that started a process of me just having to check it out.

Richard was curious about the length of time that had passed since my abuse. Was it common so much time to pass?

I explained I had learned from advocacy organizations like ChildUSA that statistically something like one-third of the victims of child sex abuse disclose as children. In most cases, I continued, this disclosure happens if and when they are caught in the act of being abused.

"Think of a situation where somebody walks in on a parent or someone else abusing a child, and either as part of that confrontation or a follow-up, the child discloses," I explained. "It is rare that a child walks out of that situation like that and tells someone about being sexually assaulted or molested on their own."

"Another one-third of the survivors of childhood sexual abuse never disclose," I told Beene. "They take that to their grave, sometimes after living a full life and dying a natural death, keeping the memory of abuse private."

"The final one-third remember later in life, like I did at the age of 44. These are the hardest cases," I told Beene. "Sometimes they drink themselves to death, overdose on drugs, or commit suicide. The effects on people who become aware of this later in life and the eventual outcome are awful."

"Suicide," Beene remarked.

I heard the word "suicide" amplified through my headphones. It startled me and delivered a grim reminder that the subject I was talking about was a matter of life and death. I took a sip of coffee and a deep breath before continuing.

I shared my perspective with Richard that I counted myself as fortunate to be in a safe, loving environment when I remembered my abuse, and that I believed that I would eventually be okay. In fact, I told him that an attorney friend whom I consulted about whether to pursue some type of civil action, mentioned that the fact that I had resources, good relationships, and an outward appearance as a guy who has his life together may make it tougher to claim any damages if I ever chose to pursue them in court.

"But many people don't have their lives together, and they end up in that middle space somewhere," I went on. "I've spoken with several people who are stuck in this sort of no-man's-land. So, it's not uncommon with children who are abused for them to wait a long time, if at all, to be able to disclose."

"Without getting too graphic, take us back to that first time you saw Dr. Zink," Richard continued. "You were injured in a baseball game, correct?"

Talking about my experience of childhood sexual abuse is difficult. The details Richard was asking about are intimate, personal. I tried to block out the image of the hundreds, or even possibly thousands, of people tuned in to their car radio or listening online at their computers, as I recounted the details of my injury and the abuse that followed. I understood that there were rules about what could or couldn't be broadcast over the air. However, I also knew that sanitizing my account of sexual abuse and molestation would not do my story justice. I needed to provide details and say the exact words that describe what happened to me to send a signal that cut through the noise of whatever else might be surrounding each listener.

"So, your father wasn't in the room fort these appointments?"

"No, not every time," I answered.

At the time, I thought that was an odd question for Richard to ask. Looking back, however, it has been a common response from others when I talk about the details of what happened to me in that first examination and the office visits that followed.

The answer I gave that my father was not in the room for every one of my medical appointments must have rung true to Richard's listeners tuning in from around Bakersfield's farming community. Even if they were not directly involved in agriculture, everyone was familiar with the seasonal ritual of independence that came with high school boys in a farming town who turned 16, got their driver's license, and quickly gained employment working for another friend's father doing manual labor for the summer: pruning grapevines, packing watermelons, moving sprinkler pipe. These were all responsibilities assigned to boys who were not yet men, but who were given the freedom to take care of themselves and their work. Driving themselves to and from the farm, the field, or the shop, without parental supervision, was not out of the ordinary for a Bakersfield kid. Neither were my solo visits to Zink. What he did to me, however, was anything but ordinary.

"When you look back on that, do you ever remember a time when the sixteen-or seventeen-year-old version of yourself said this is not right, I need to tell someone. Did you even consider that?"

"No," I answered.

"If you think about the culture at the time," I told Beene, "doctors were people of authority. Whether it was another parent or a teacher or a coach or a pastor or a doctor, those folks in my world anyway had higher priority status. For me to experience something uncomfortable at a doctor's office wasn't necessarily uncommon, but to have something like this happen, I don't know if I could make sense of it. So those were likely my first thoughts about the experience."

I told Beene that I knew when I went away to college, and eventually when I moved away as an adult, that I wasn't going to go back and see this guy.

"I felt like the things that were done to me were unusual enough that they were wrong," I said. "But to be honest with you, life moved on. These were extremely uncomfortable experiences, so burying them and in many ways trying to forget about them by either drinking or using drugs was my playbook during my young adult years because it didn't feel like something that I even had the ability or the language to tell anybody about."

"Dr. Zink was actually charged, and there was a trial, right? You were gone when he went on trial right? You weren't party to that matter?"

"Yes," I answered. "Zink was charged in the spring of 1994, followed by a trial in the early summer that same year."

I told Beene that I had no recollection of this, probably because I was away at college at the time. There was barely an internet and no social media, therefore I wasn't as tuned in to what was happening in my hometown on a day-to-day basis as I might be now.

"Jeff, I want to get this right. You didn't know about his trial until 2017 when you were talking to your wife." Beene asked, "is that correct?"

I went on to tell Beene about the first time I remembered my abuse in the fall of 2017. I told him that reading the details of the charges against Zink, and the descriptions of abuse provided by each of the boy defendants, gave me certainty that my memory was accurate. The things they were describing in the articles were exactly what I remembered happening to me.

"With this certainty, however, came days and weeks of hell," I said. "I felt as if I was experiencing the trauma all over again, triggering feelings of extreme shame, sadness, and panic attacks, which I had never experienced before."

"What was that like? What was going through your mind?"

I told Beene that Stephanie described it initially as just tremendously sad.

"Imagine the person you love the most in your life," I went on, "whether your spouse or your children, telling you something that was just buried forever, causing suffering, extremely painful in the moment. I was tearful; she was empathetic. Probably for days, if not weeks afterward, I cried myself to sleep just not being able to make sense of what the heck happened to me and how it could have happened so clearly with others, and nothing had been done."

"In the weeks that followed, interestingly, I experienced more than just the sadness that comes along with these types of memories," I said.

With the images of Zink's face fresh in my mind, I told Beene about the charity event and my first panic attack. I spoke about leaving the event and thinking that I didn't want to die and interrupt the charity event honoring the dedicated volunteer service of this wonderful man who bore such a striking resemblance to Zink but was not in fact him. Very Catholic of me. How screwed up is that?

"At that point after about a week or so of being upset and having similar incidents," I explained, "I knew I needed to get help, talk to a doctor and figure out some way to stabilize my emotions while I could make sense of all of this."

"So then what did you do?"

I told Beene and his listeners about my efforts to pursue criminal and administrative justice, and about the frustrating experience of running into dead ends caused by the various statutes of limitations. There were various steps I could take by filing official statements with the Orlando Police or the Florida Board of Medicine, but in both cases the doctor who abused me as a child would be notified. I had no idea what this man was capable of and was somewhat afraid of what he might do if he knew I was the person filing the complaint. It was really frightening to think about.

As for handling this as a civil matter, I told Beene that I had reviewed Florida statues for these specific crimes. Then I called a friend of mine who is an experienced attorney in medical malpractice. On its own, even if I reported this closer to the date of the crime, because it was something the doctor would have claimed as a bona fide medical procedure, it gets complicated. When you remember it later as a repressed memory like I did, however, the statute of limitations is tolled – essentially suspended – and begins on the date that you remember. Proving this, however, is extremely difficult. With this understanding, I just was not sure that I wanted to pursue this in civil court. While it certainly was not about the money, however, I did want justice.

I told Beene that I decided that what I needed to do was gather more information. That would involve talking to the hospital system where Zink was on staff. Sometime in the summer of 2018, I wrote letters to the president of the hospital system and the doctor who was president of the medical staff. I never heard from either of them directly, but I did receive a letter from the risk management department saying that while they were sorry for what had happened to me, the incidents did not occur on their watch. They were unable and unwilling to assist me in my effort to pursue revocation of Zink's medical license.

"A year and a half later, in January of 2020, I reached out directly to the corporation's CEO via LinkedIn and email. There was no follow-up. Nothing was done."

"At the very least," I explained, "I expected the CEO to listen. I expected the CEO to use his voice and state that practicing medicine in his hospital system is a privilege, and one that can be revoked. I believe the information I provided was enough for the CEO to make a business decision or a mission decision. However, just having a conversation would have felt like I was heard."

"Don't get me wrong. I run a business, and I am not so naïve to believe that there is no calculus that the hospital system applies when reviewing complaints like mine. They must determine whether I am a wingnut or if I have a legitimate concern. Either way, however, businesses like this hospital system still have to understand that people want to be heard."

"What do you mean by that?" Beene asked. "Talk about the reluctance of victims to come forward for fear that they won't be heard or that they will be dismissed."

"At its very basic level," I explained, "child sex abuse is a trauma. Your brain works in a way that its initial response, its instinct if you will, is to try to protect yourself. Your brain does all sorts of things to do that, whether it buries it forever, or for a time, in my case 30 years. Eventually when it did come out, I went through a period trying to make sure that my memory was correct and that the things I remembered were accurate. This was supported by my own research."

"My other instinct, however, was to protect the other people around me that I love. This doesn't make sense logically and requires some explanation. I shared my story with Stephanie, who thankfully was empathetic and heard me and basically let me talk and share my pain and suffering. Along the way, the few people who I was able to share this with from a clinical perspective . . . my doctor, my therapist, a few very close friends who are doctors as well . . . along with a few surfing buddies who stand shoulder to shoulder with me on this, my instinct was to keep it in until I was able to make sense about what this is going to do for my life and understand what I was able to do with it going forward.

"This tendency to be in control probably comes as no surprise. I was a CEO in Bakersfield and am a CEO in my current job; in high school I was a catcher, captain of the team. I'm a recovering control freak but I still like to be in charge. If there was one thing that I was going to be darn sure about with this, it was that I was going to be in charge about how it affected me going forward. So, sharing it with others kind of potentially puts you at risk because you really don't know how people are doing to respond. You read all sorts of stories about people not being believed or dismissed or having to prove it. So as long as I was going to be able to control how this rolled out, I was going to keep my cards very close. So that meant keeping this very private until I found myself with enough information and the experience of going through the steps to pursue justice until all other options were exhausted. Then I decided it was time to go public."

"Why did you decide to deal with this way you did? Writing blog?"

"I am a very private person," I told Beene. "In spite of my public job, I take the privacy of my friends, family, and business colleagues very seriously. I did not want to blast this out or spill it out over a dinner or something like that and really impose on the busy lives of friends or family or others. I gave some thought and wondered if I was on the receiving end of this, what would be the simplest way to receive it, digest it, and take time to drink it in? I came up with my method of sending a simple email each day, essentially one chapter at a time, something that was easy to read over cup of coffee or in between meetings, rather than book or long form article.

The timeframe I chose to distribute it began with the 30th anniversary of my abuse and lasted for 18 days. Eighteen is symbolic in Judaism. It represents the Hebrew word chai, which means life. Writing and sending this out each day has been a meditation for me and hopefully for those who are reading it.

What happened to me was wrong, but I still have a lot of life to live," I said. "I can do something to help myself to heal. I can do something that can possibly help others to do the same. I can fight for justice."

As the interview wound up, I imagined some of my dearest friends from Bakersfield listening in. Tung, the Vietnamese head and neck cancer surgeon who was also my neighbor, would be wrapping up his busy day of taking care of patients, remembering the night I told him and his wife, Ingrid, my story after our children were asleep following a long day of skiing on Christmas break. Herb, the Bakersfield native and local newspaper writer, would be finishing up his latest column, perhaps about a recent surfing trip, a concert, or the banalities of life in the Central Valley. John, the Riverside native and pioneering citrus farmer, would be in his truck on the edge of a grove, watching the last of the Cara Cara Navel oranges being picked. There would be many others, too.

I also imagined strangers as angels and airwaves drifted into their homes, to soothe an ache, to dry a tear, to quell a rage triggered by memories of their own "Dr. Zinks." Boys who had become men. Men who had become fathers. Fathers who had trauma of their own, cut from the same cloth as mine.

I shared my story, with a little help from my friends. It has been my way to let other people in, follow along, be a part of it and use common threads to mend the torn fabric in their own lives.

25
Telling My Parents

Deciding how and when to tell my parents about my childhood sexual abuse was one of the biggest struggles for me throughout the whole process.

My family is close. I have two younger brothers and we have been nearly inseparable since childhood, if not by physical proximity, then by any other way possible. As a parent myself, I knew I was going to be telling my own parents something that would probably break their hearts. At the end of the day, choosing to share something that could break my mother's and father's hearts was just not a choice I wanted to make on any day on any topic. I held that one closely until I knew I was going to go public and share my story.

Beginning in 2019, Sunday mornings had taken on a different routine from the Catholic tradition I practiced during Colin and Olivia's grade-school and middle-school years. Stephanie was raised Jewish, and with our youngest son, Grant, in kindergarten, my Sunday routine was driving him and his best friend, Ari, to Sunday school at the Temple.

After waving goodbye to the boys, I had a few hours to myself before picking them up. I drove to the beach and found a spot with some shade and a breeze. It was a few days before the 30th anniversary of my abuse.

I called my parents, and my dad answered. I wished him good morning and gave him the Vero Beach surf report. He told me that they were in the car, driving to the beach themselves, a couple of hours up the Atlantic coast. After catching up for a while, I cast a look out onto the tourmaline sea and felt its gentle tug. It was time.

I breathed a heavy sigh. After a fumbled apology for what I was about to say, I told my dad and mom that I needed to share some difficult news with them. I told them about Dr. Zink, his abuse, how and when I remembered, and what the past couple of years had been like. I kept my composure for the most part, until a feeling of sadness began to well up from somewhere deep inside me.

They didn't say anything. The phone was silent for almost a full minute, but it seemed like an eternity. Then they wondered out loud about why I was telling them this now and not sooner.

Knowing that all of this could have caused my parents a lot of pain and potentially some guilt, I told them that once I remembered this for the first time in the Fall of 2017, I just made an adult decision keep from telling them for as long as I could. I didn't want to hurt them.

My dad was curious to know if I had talked to my brothers or anyone else who had similar experiences. I did not know other patients of Zink's personally, but I told him that I had read about others who had come forward in his trial. As for Jason and Joel, I told my dad I did what I had always done as their older brother. I tried to protect them. I checked with each of my younger brothers to see if anything like what I remembered ever happened to them since they each had seen Dr. Zink following their own sports-related injuries. Nothing as severe as what I had reported was in their memories – just recollections of Zink's odd bedside manner and memories of visits to his office that were uncomfortable for them as children.

"We thought we asked you about Dr. Zink," my mom said. "We were aware of the allegations, but we talked to each of you boys and checked it out."

I told my parents that it is possible that I repressed that memory or that I was so embarrassed and ashamed that I did not want to tell them. I told them that I have no resentments about the way they have dealt (or not dealt) with this issue over the last 30 years. I told them I did not want to burden them, but that the time had come for me to tell them as I was preparing to go public with my story in a few days.

I told my dad and mom that the only person that I believe is at fault is Dr. William P. Zink. That I believe he is a serial sex abuser of children who got away with his crimes. He was very manipulative – as manipulative as someone can get – by currying favor with our family, endearing himself to us, and stepping in at a very vulnerable time in my life when all I cared about was getting healthy and returning to the baseball field. It was all that my parents wanted, too. Like a master, Zink was able to take advantage of that and use that as an opportunity for 18 months to sexually abuse me.

I believe that there is a primal instinct inside every parent to protect their children. While my parents are in their seventies, and my brothers and I are all in our forties, I am certain that my story triggered that instinct inside my dad and mom.

I also believe that my parents probably felt some sense of responsibility, maybe shame. As I have listened to parents of others whose own children reported childhood sexual abuse, there is this seed of guilt that never goes away. It is truly heartbreaking to hear.

I told my dad and mom that it was likely that they may receive inquiries from other friends and family who read what I planned to share publicly. If they did, I suggested that they respond by telling people that they did not know, that they love and support me, and that I would be willing to take any calls or emails to answer questions that they were not able to answer. I told them I did not expect them to answer for me, and was only asking for their love and support.

In my radio interview with Richard Beene, he asked me if I thought by not telling my parents I was somehow saving them. I told him that I thought it was important to protect anyone who might be harmed just by knowing my story and the terrible experience that I had gone through. My parents fell into that category.

That is the same message I sent to my mom sometime during the following week of February 13, 2020, in response to a text I received from her after my story went public. The tone of her text sounded surprised, even though I had informed her about my plan to start sharing my story publicly online.

My reply was not received well. The text message I received back from my mom did not make me feel heard. It made me feel ashamed.

Dad and I are very sorry learning about what you had to go through. We thought we did our due diligence years ago. Through all your visits, in surgery and appointments, we never observed any questionable practice by the doctor. That said, Dad and I are very concerned and hurt that over the past two years when you've consulted with other people, and even over the past 30 years, you would not have the confidence to share with us what you were going through. We were very hurt to learn about it at the end of a phone conversation and a written blog which you have obviously contemplated for a long time. We are heartbroken that we did not realize the abuse. It cuts us to our core. We are very sorry, but we are also hurt that you would not confide in us while you confided in attorneys and others. We are your family. Why did you eliminate us from the initial conversations? We are fielding phone calls and we have no answers because we were unaware. We are very sorry, but we feel very blindsided and unable to even comprehend.

My mom's response fractured our relationship and caused me great pain. I could not respond. Stephanie did so for me, advocating for what I needed.

The following Sunday, my dad drove down from Orlando to Vero Beach to meet for breakfast. His presence was comforting, but his inability to understand that my decision to proceed the way I did was about me and not about Mom or him was too much. Despite time and several attempts over the years to repair this fracture, the distance between us remains a source of great pain.

I believe there is a reason why we have parents. Not the biological reason, it is more existential. We have parents because we are so vulnerable as children that we need protection from bad things happening to us. To survive this trauma, I still did.

I am forever grateful to Stephanie for assuming this role of defender and advocate that neither of us ever likely considered when we said our wedding vows. She is my rock and my strength – always, and especially through the challenges that were still ahead of me.

26
Telling My Children

With our youngest child, Grant, I did not tell him anything. He was five years old in February of 2020, and I just did not believe that there was anything about my experience that was appropriate to share with him, or that he would even understand. However, we have had age-appropriate conversations about personal space, appropriate touch, and what type of contact is allowed by other people.

With our two older children, Colin and Olivia, we have an open door for communication with them. They were in high school and are mature enough to discuss most adult topics. As very young children, when they were ages 4 and 5, they had already heard me share the worst news possible . . . that my wife and their birth mother, Debby, had died. It was the hardest thing I have ever had to do, and I am sure the most difficult news they have every received. They survived and have thrived since. I knew they would be able to handle what I was about to tell them.

A day or so before I went public, Stephanie and I sat down with them at the dining room table of the townhome we were renting until our new home on the island was ready for us to move in. I told them that I had some difficult news to share.

I told them that I had been dealing with some memories of a traumatic experience from my childhood and that they needed to know. I walked them through general details of my abuse and told them that I buried it and that my parents (their grandparents) were not aware until the previous weekend. I apologized to them for being somewhat distant during the prior year, but that this was something that seriously affected me during that period and that I was getting help from my doctor and a therapist.

By this time, I had gotten better about making myself vulnerable. This was a different kind of vulnerability, however, being displayed in front of my children. I am their dad, their protector, and as soon as the words started to come out of my mouth, I dreaded the idea of this setting – a rented townhouse on the Florida mainland, miles from the familiar, comforting ocean – as their memory. I am glad we do not live there anymore.

Both children were very empathetic and loving in their responses. Olivia, was emotional at first, but she is also headstrong – very Irish. I could see the fire in her eyes, wanting to do something to defend me, to right this wrong. Colin is more sensitive. He really internalized what I told him. Seeing the pain in my son's eyes, observing him realize for the first time in his young life that I am not invincible, was hard.

When I decided to go public, I kept a journal of what helped. In addition to Stephanie's love and support, Colin and Olivia's support and understanding were number two on the list.

I cannot remember a time in my life when I felt more vulnerable than when I told my children. Out of all people, how they managed to respond the way they did defines what it means to experience grace.

For anyone who may find themselves in the same situation, where someone tells you that they were sexually abused, I strongly encourage centering a response around the ideas and these words:

I believe you.

I love you and support you.

I will be here for you as you go through this.

Any iteration of that can help any survivor of childhood sexual abuse to heal and can lead toward a path of recovery.

27
Guidance for Healing, Talking to a Therapist

have shared publicly that I lost my first wife, Debby, to alcoholism. She was my first soulmate and mother to my two older children, Colin and Olivia. While we were divorced at the time of her death, an action I took to protect myself and my children, I grieved the loss of a friend, a spouse, and a loving mother. A skilled therapist helped me to heal.

When Stephanie and I fell in love, I was a single father raising two young children on my own. She accepted me unconditionally, and I believe my children saw the truth in her love. They fell in love with her and she with them. We were married and she eventually adopted Colin and Olivia, becoming their "mommy on earth." After much consideration by the entire family, Stephanie and I decided to have a child of our own. A son was born. We named him Grant, which means "gift." Again, a skilled therapist helped me to trust myself, to trust Stephanie, and to trust the new family we formed together.

Having an individual therapist to turn to, talk to, and to guide me through the process of recovering from the trauma of childhood sexual abuse has been critical. So has group therapy with other adult men survivors. Family and friends cannot shoulder this.

Before asking for help, I was a cliché. In my mind, asking for help with my personal problems was something that I associated with weakness. Depending on someone else to do something for me, rather than do it for myself, was unbecoming. There were and still are a lot of societal influences that deter victims of childhood sexual abuse from reaching out for help. They are an illusion, made up and made stronger by perpetual silence.

My therapists are in my corner. Individual therapy has helped me to sort through the memories, to acknowledge my abuse, to have compassion for the boy who was abused, and to have empathy for the man who remembered it. Group therapy has helped me to recognize unhealthy or unhelpful coping methods and to make better choices. Both forms of therapy have helped me to stop feeling guilty about standing up for myself. They have helped me find the courage to speak out and seek justice for myself and others.

Asking for help was nearly impossible for me, until it wasn't. Being helped allowed me to experience another type of grace that I hope to never forget. Ultimately, I did the work, but therapy made it possible.

28

The Human Brain After the Trauma of Childhood Sexual Abuse

There have been several periods of time since remembering my childhood sexual assault by Dr. Zink that I struggled to understand why I never prevented or stopped him from doing what he did to me. Initially, I settled on the notion that I was simply being compliant, following the lead of someone who I knew and trusted and who was acting in my best interest. Over time, however, as I began to remember more details about the various times I was subjected to even more and more abuse, this notion did not sit right with me.

I still could not understand how a bookish, gangly, rather unimposing man was able to overpower me and do what he did without me fighting back. By the time of my last and worst abuse by Dr. Zink, I was eighteen years old, five feet ten inches tall and weighed 180 pounds. I could bench press 275 pounds and I could run two miles in under thirteen minutes.

In addition to the knee injury that Zink was treating me for, as a teenager I had suffered and recovered from a shoulder injury from an awkward throw, a broken nose from a collision with a pitcher while chasing a pop-up in foul territory, and countless broken fingers and toes from foul-tipped balls. I was a tough kid, but for some reason I did not defend myself against Zink. After remembering my sexual abuse, there was a period when I could not forgive myself for what I believed was something that I could have prevented or stopped.

According to an article that appeared in a 2014 edition of Time which summarized a report prepared for Harvard Medical School, James Hopper, Ph.D. and David Lisak, Ph.D. stated that "In the midst of a sexual assault, the brain's fear circuitry takes over while other key parts are impaired or even effectively shutting down. This is the brain reacting to a life-threatening situation just the way it is supposed to do."

While I find no comfort in the memory of being sexually abused by Dr. Zink as a child, I have found solace in the perspectives of Drs. Hopper and Lisak. The abuse was not my fault. I was powerless. To survive, my brain did what it was supposed to do.

The work of Dr. Rebecca Campbell, Professor of Psychology at Michigan State University, has also helped me. Her writing and teaching about the neurobiology of trauma helped me by providing a clinical understanding of the brain and how it responds to trauma. Her research is the proof I need when feelings of doubt arise about whether there was anything that I could have done to respond to my abuse, or for that matter, even remember it until it was safe to do so.

In the face of fear, safety measures made possible by the cerebrum, prefrontal cortex, amygdala, and hypothalamus all worked together. Oxytocin, catecholamine, adrenaline, and cortisol were released. Fight or flight, or in my case a state of tonic immobility were the possible results. The interconnected functions of these various parts of the brain and chemicals are the result of thousands of years of evolutionary adaptations that were beyond my control. These ancient responses kept me alive. Knowing that gives me a sense of peace.

As for the repression of the memory, I believe my brain did what smart brains do. It packed away the trauma until it was safe for the memory to come out. Fortunately for me it was in the loving presence of someone like my wife. I realize that I am fortunate that the environment was right for me, and I empathize with other victims whose time and circumstance for healing never comes.

29

One Small Step, February 27, 2020

After 30 years of silence, and more than two years of unsuccessful efforts to pursue criminal, administrative, and civil justice for being sexually assaulted and molested by Dr. William P. Zink, on the morning of February 27, 2020, the "Find Doctors" function on the AdventHealth for Children website read "No Results" when searching for Dr. Zink's name. I tried the search again and imagined the following algorithms at work.

Dr. William P. Zink + 18 months of sexual abuse + 30 years of silence + 16 blog chapters emailed to friends and family + 10 posts on Advent-Health social media sites on 02/26/2020 + 1 radio interview + social media doing its thing = No Results on AdventHealth for Children's Website.

A Search for Dr. William P. Zink on AdventHealth for Children's Website = No Results.

Dr. William P. Zink = Nothing.

In 1853, the abolitionist minister Theodore Parker delivered a sermon and said "I do not pretend to understand the moral universe. The arc is a long one. My eye reaches but little ways. I cannot calculate the curve and complete the figure by experience of sight. I can divine it by conscience. And from what I see I am sure it bends toward justice."

The incremental justice of seeing Dr. Zink's headshot and contact information removed from AdventHealth's website does not appear as a right angle. Instead, it is subtle, likely made possible by an anonymous engineer deleting one or two lines of code. If one was not paying attention, it might even be overlooked entirely. After recording a radio interview about my story that morning, followed by an entire day's worth of social media posts making the rounds referencing AdventHealth's website pages, even I did not receive notification that the change was made. It just happened.

And while I am grateful that the risk of an unsuspecting parent booking a pediatric orthopedic appointment with Dr. Zink for their injured child through AdventHealth's website is gone, I still wonder "What took so long?" I may never find out, but if I am ever invited to share my perspective about how AdventHealth might improve their response to someone like me, I will encourage their leadership to use more empathy and less risk management if they truly want to demonstrate their commitment to extending the healing ministry of Christ. Actually, it is a point of view I would be glad to share with any institution that is serious about changing the way the respond to and manage information of such a sensitive nature.

As for Dr. William P. Zink, continuing to operate and see patients, according to his own website, he is still practicing. According to the state of Florida, his medical license remains in good standing despite complaints requesting its revocation.

While he must be near retirement, if surgery remains part of his practice, he will likely need to affiliate with another healthcare system or stand-alone surgery center. People will find out which ones, and hopefully share what they know about my experience of being sexually abused and molested by him as a child. These organizations will have to make their own decisions about whether they want to affiliate with him or not.

I imagine someday, the steady stream of patients that Dr. Zink has relied on to earn his living will dry up. He will probably retire, close his practice, and someday he will die.

Ben Gibbard of the indie-rock band, Death Cab for Cutie, wrote the song "I Will Follow You into the Dark" which perfectly describes what I imagine a monster like Zink might find as he exhales his final breath. Heaven and Hell may decide that they both are satisfied. They will illuminate the "NO" on their vacancy signs. It will be dark for eternity, without a hint of a spark—the blackest of rooms.

30
Feel (W)hole

"Feel Whole." Two words I read on street signs on the afternoon of March 6, 2020, when I arrived for a meeting called by AdventHealth following the publication of my story. The request from the corporation's legal department was that I come in to meet to discuss a "solution that works for you, and us, and the community."

As I entered the lobby, I wondered which one of AdventHealth's CEO's, Terry Shaw or Darryl Tol, signed off on the marketing campaign using the words "Feel Whole," knowing since 2018, that a member of the medical staff repeatedly sexually assaulted me as a child by putting his ungloved finger in my rectum on multiple occasions while treating me for a knee injury? Feel Whole? Feel Hole? Surely these two gentlemen must know about homophones.

"Feel Whole." The words were stretched across banners in the lobby of the organization's executive office building in downtown Orlando, right underneath the organization's mission of "Extending the healing ministry of Christ." Now I've read the Bible passage where Jesus licked his fingers and stuck them in the ears of a deaf man to restore his hearing, but this might be a stretch.

"Feel Whole." Two words next to AdventHealth's logotype that quickly evoked the image of the headshot of Dr. William P. Zink I found when Googling his name in the fall of 2017, when I remembered the repressed memory of being sexually assaulted and molested as a child by him under the guise of medical care 30 years ago.

Heart racing. Brow sweating. Room spinning. Wondering if this was a mistake.

"With a personalized greeting like that, who wouldn't feel welcome?" came a booming voice from across the lobby. I turned to see the smiling face of my childhood friend and local Orlando attorney, Michael Scoma, who agreed to join me for this meeting. "They probably should have run that one by someone with a 13-year old's sense of humor before spending millions to plaster it all over town," he said. "Idiots. Let's go see what they have to say."

Walking into the executive conference room at AdventHealth's headquarters, I was immediately grateful for my decision to bring a friend as I was met by four people – a health system executive, a member of the legal department, outside counsel, and the organization's new president of the medical staff ... who used to be my own primary care doctor. For a moment, I thought that this was the ultimate mind-screw and hoped that this was just an odd coincidence.

Curiously absent from this meeting were the two people I had contacted in 2018 and 2020: AdventHealth CEO, Terry Shaw, and AdventHealth Central Florida CEO, Daryl Tol. If the priest and the Levite couldn't make the meeting, I was hoping that at least one of the people in the room would be the Good Samaritan I needed to hear from. Beyond the kindness expressed by my old doctor, I would have no such luck.

After exchanging pleasantries, I was asked to offer my perspective about what this reluctant cabal could do to help. "I was thinking you might be able to tell me, since you called the meeting," I responded.

Nobody answered my request. We sat in silence for a full minute.

Sensing my frustration, my attorney shot me a knowing Jedi-mind-trick glance and gave me a nod, prompting the following:

"What is the business purpose for AdventHealth maintaining a relationship with Dr. Zink?" I asked.

"It's complicated," they replied, followed by a longwinded explanation of the bylaws and rules governing relationships with medical staff, versus the contracts maintained with members of the medical group, the division of authority between corporate and legal and the medical staff, and medical staff credentialing. Luckily both Stephanie and I grew up in medical households and had prior work experience in healthcare philanthropy, so I had a basic understanding of this byzantine arrangement designed to protect corporate assets, doctors' egos, and hopefully, a few patients along the way. Frankly, this all sounded like bureaucratic bullshit, with no hint of common sense.

"How long has Dr. Zink been on the medical staff?" I asked.

"Since the 1980's," they answered.

"What is the average annual revenue that AdventHealth makes from a pediatric orthopedic surgeon who is credentialed and given privileges to perform surgery in one of your hospitals?" I asked.

"I do not know that number off hand," the president of the medical staff replied.

I asked the same question of the health system executive who responded, "Well, leaving money out of it, a busy pediatric orthopedic surgeon probably performs around 400 surgeries annually. Dr. Zink was probably performing ten percent of that volume in the last year."

Ten percent of 400. That's 40 patients each year during the two years since I contacted Terry Shaw and Daryl Tol. 80 kids. Statistics are that one out of every six of these children will be sexually assaulted before they turn eighteen years old. That's thirteen kids treated by Dr. William P. Zink between 2018 and 2020 who, statistically speaking, may be victims of sexual assault.

If I were CEO of AdventHealth, would I take a chance that thirteen kids who received surgery in my hospital system would be introduced to a guy whose public reputation from a Google search would not qualify him as a volunteer for the public library or the babysitting service offered by the local church? Hell, no. But it's complicated.

Before attending this meeting, I ran my questions by a few friends. Some had experience in healthcare, and others were just hardworking businesspeople with years of tough decisions under their belts. I tested two of the observations out on the crowd gathered in the conference room.

"One buddy of mine suggested his perception that this is purely about business and money. Zink is 'damaged goods' and AdventHealth can get him to perform surgery for as little as they can and keep the spread between what they pay him and what they bill insurance," I offered.

"Absolutely not," the health system executive protested. "I know Terry Shaw and Daryl Tol, and I can assure you that they are good men who would never put money before patient safety or quality," a breathless reply before she had to excuse herself from this important meeting to go catch an airplane.

"Another buddy of mine suggested his perception that this might have more to do with the organization's faith-based mission. Perhaps they are trying to show forgiveness and give Zink a second chance," I suggested.

The president of the medical staff spoke up and offered what I find to be the one noble point of view of the whole meeting. "My number one priority is patient care and safety," he said. "While there are bylaws and rules, I can assure you that your story will be considered the next time Dr. Zink's petition for privileges is reviewed. Nothing about what you've shared aligns with our mission of extending the healing ministry of Christ."

I might have been satisfied to end there, but the outside counsel chimed in with an odd request. "Perhaps you might help us by encouraging the few people who you have heard from since publishing your story to come forward and file their own complaint?"

Do you mean the busy mom who contacted me after reading about my story on social media who told me about the time when her son was injured in a weekend sporting event a few years prior? Dr. Zink offered to pick her son up in his own car to drive to an exam on a Sunday. "While it was creepy," she said to me, "I don't think it qualifies as abuse." No, it's called grooming.

Or do you mean the childhood friend who lives out of the country and has more than a decade of recovery from alcoholism and cocaine addiction under his belt who called me on Sunday after reading my blog? Dr. Zink drugged and raped him in his medical office when he was 14 years old. "I called to tell you I am glad that you are telling your story," he said to me. "My recovery requires that I leave that in the past. I am healing, one day at a time, and all I want to put into the world is my art and love." I respect that, my brother. I love you.

"Feel Whole." It probably started as a good idea, hoping to inspire thoughts of healing body, mind, and spirit while under the care of AdventHealth and its medical staff. I can picture the white-board session now, an echo chamber of adulation. A zippy video with images of healthy people doing healthy things backed by a soundtrack and a final coda call-and-response of "Tell me how you're feeling tonight." Hashtagwordcloud #feelingwhole fade to AdventHealthlogo.

Statistically speaking, it is likely that there is a mom or dad in the Orlando area who saw that video on social media somewhere. It made them feel good. It evoked a sense of trust in AdventHealth, a trusted resource that a parent should be able to rely on for a referral to a doctor who will help their child feel whole.

Not Feel (W)hole.

NOT FEEL (W)HOLE.

31

Zink Quits, No Longer Affiliated with AdventHealth

When I began my journey to recover and heal from the trauma of childhood sexual abuse by my doctor, my mission was to seek justice and help others by sharing my story. At the time, I believed that the easiest step would be reporting Dr. William P. Zink to the healthcare system where he was on medical staff so that his hospital privileges would be revoked. Little did I know that this would be one of the hardest parts of my journey.

On the evening of March 13, 2020, however, I received a phone call from a senior officer of the corporation reporting that Dr. Zink resigned from the medical staff, and that he is no longer affiliated with Advent-Health. I do not know if it was pressure from my emails, his peers, the hospital administration, or the universe, but the bottom line is Dr. Zink quit. I felt overwhelming relief, but surprisingly I also felt empathy for the various people like my old primary care doctor, the new medical staff president that had been pulled into this unpleasant experience along the way. Thankfully he was there, but regretfully he was also burdened.

After reporting the facts, the caller said that my visit to Advent-Health's executive office on Friday March 6th and the details of my story started AdventHealth's leadership on a journey that arrived at the destination of Zink's resignation. I expressed gratitude for the news. I also shared my point of view that the pain and suffering caused by the inaction of AdventHealth CEO Terry Shaw and AdventHealth Central Florida CEO Daryl Tol over the past two years was unnecessary and entirely avoidable had they demonstrated better leadership and exercised better judgement by responding to my concerns sooner rather than later. I said that two years is a long time to sit and wait for the phone to ring, wondering all the while if another 16-year-old boy operated on by Dr. Zink in an AdventHealth hospital was being fondled, or photographed in the nude, or worse, at his follow up appointments in Zink's private office.

And then it happened, with the very next words spoken by the caller from AdventHealth. "I know it may seem simple," the caller said, "but there really are complicated bylaws and rules that don't allow the company CEOs to have more than one vote each on the board that oversees the credentialing process that gives doctors privileges to practice in our hospitals. We do try really hard. It's just not that easy."

I was being gaslighted.

I heard the faintest tinkly, jangly sound in my ears. I started to feel a floaty, drifty dissociation. I could hear the caller saying words that were crystal clear, but they seemed to propel me out into the weightless dark.

I was a 46-year-old grown man, a married father of three, with a 25-year career in philanthropy who is CEO of a $100 million dollar company, and I was being manipulated to see it their way. This was "no, but" in full force. "Yes, and" were nowhere to be seen.

I heard it again, but louder. A tinkly, jangly sound in my ears. I was floating, drifting, dissociating.

I pictured my oldest son, just weeks away from his 16th birthday. The same age that I was when Dr. Zink first stuck his ungloved finger in my ass. The same age I was when Dr. Zink held my balls in his bare hands. The same age I was when Dr. Zink turned out the lights, pulled down my pants and took dirty pictures of me as a boy while whispering "lower, lower" until he could see my teenage dick.

I was filling with rage. I pictured the childhood friend of mine, who called when he had read my blog after I started sharing my story, to tell me that two years before my own sexual assault, when he was just 14, that he was bent over an examination table and fucked in the ass by Dr. Zink. He told me that he was drugged and raped by Dr. Zink while his dad ran errands during a Saturday morning office visit. He told me that he spent his twenties guzzling gallons of booze and snorting piles of coke just to forget the scent of Dr. Zink's aftershave. Drugging and raping unsuspecting children. This is what Zink was capable of.

The rage consumed me.

Was this caller trying to persuade me to see the other side, to understand the reasons behind their initial answer of "it's complicated"? How could the bearer of such good news be so smug, so obtuse? A hot rod sycophant angling for a better spot in the corporate pecking order of AdventHealth. Hardheaded, not hearing me, no empathy. Silently, I repelled him by channeling the seething rage the late, great Chris Cornell delivered in Soundgarden's 1997 punk rock thrash "Ty Cobb."

Sick in the head, sick in the mouth,
Can't hear a word you say.

Not a bit, and I don't give a shit.
I got the glass, I got the steel, I got everything
All I need is your head on a stake.
Hard headed fuck you all
Hard headed fuck you all
Hard headed fuck you all
Just add it up to the hot rod death toll.

That night, under pressure, Dr. William P. Zink quit the medical staff and is no longer affiliated with AdventHealth. That is a good thing, and something worth celebrating.

However, Zink was still operating a private practice in Orlando, accepting insurance payments from most major insurers and many large self-insured employers in Florida. Who knows where he will perform surgery, but he can still see children in his own private office.

I wondered what else I, or anyone, could do to stop him? I checked my insurance policy, and Zink was listed in the network for referrals. I contacted my benefits administrator and asked to have him removed.

Zink is also still licensed by the State of Florida to practice medicine. While numerous complaints have been filed, given the State Board of Medicine's reluctance to discipline one of their own, it may never come of anything. I am not satisfied but know that at least I have done my part.

Many people played a part in the small victory of Zink being forced to resign from AdventHealth's medical staff. There is more work to be done, and I will stick with it.

Zink will quit. I won't.

32
In Repair, March 15-31, 2020

On March 15, 2020, at 4:28a.m., the universe sent me a gift. Before 4:28a.m. on March 15, 2020, the last time I remember listening to John Mayer's 2006 album Continuum was in 2008. Specifically, I remember listening to the song "In Repair" sometime between the day Debby died and the day I fell in love with Stephanie. I remember putting on headphones and taking one of the longest, coldest walks of my life along the Chicago lakefront. A single father of two, contemplating my future.

The song begins with a Hammond organ played through a whirring Leslie amplifier. Then it winds its way through the first verse, a bridge, and the skipped heartbeat thump of the chorus, "I am ... in repair. I am ... in repair." Second verse, bridge, and again the skipped heartbeat thump of the chorus, "I am ... (thump thump) in repair. I am ... (thump thump) in repair." Then a slow-hand guitar solo, all at once aping Buddy Guy, channeling Allman Brothers tone. Third verse, bridge and a crescendo to the outro call-and-response, "I'm in repair. I'm not together, but I'm getting there."

At 4:28a.m. on March 15, 2020, the universe clicked on my bedside speaker and played that song. Thirty years of silence, two years of pursuing justice and a Friday evening hashmark in the "win" column in a season that is not over yet. But for 45 minutes, I laid quietly in bed listening to a cosmic gift of a 10-song iTunes playlist that seems just about right for where I am in the world right now, but also for where the world is in me.

- "In Repair" – John Mayer
- "Down the Line" – Jose Gonzales
- "Money Saves" – Delta Spirit
- "Neighbor" – Band of Horses
- "Ojala Pudiera Borrarte" – Mana
- "No Moon" – Iron and Wine

- "Happiness Loves Company" – Red Hot Chili Peppers
- "Funky Miracle" – Bonerama
- "Shelter You Through" – Andrew Duhon
- "Blood Test" – Kris Delmhorst

For several weeks I had been "making" something by publishing my story at www.stillpracticingmetoo.fyi and putting it out into the universe. At 4.28a.m. on March 15, 2020, the universe and its benevolent algorithm "made" something and returned the favor. With the world facing a pandemic, the country in a state of emergency and the prospect of at least two weeks of kids out of school, I took this as a sign, permission in fact, to unplug and use the uncertainty of the weeks that followed to "make" some more.

Make amends, make art, make dinner, make good, make jokes, make love, make a mess, make music, make nice, make no little plans for they have no magic to stir men's blood, make out, make rain, make sense, make time, make waves.

I encourage anyone going through a period of healing and recovery, if they are so inclined, to keep track of what you "make" during that time. Whatever it is, the world will be better for it.

33
One Giant Leap, July 1, 2020

In Florida and most states across the country, the practice of medicine is a privilege granted by the state. One might even call it a sacred privilege; a gentle balance between the art and science of giving life, promoting healing, and eventually witnessing death with dignity.

In Florida, the process for filing a complaint against a medical doctor with the Board of Medicine is a complicated and daunting task that I believe is challenging for the most stable, capable people. Once filed, a complaint is investigated by the Florida Department of Health and follows an enforcement process whose absurd complexity can only be illustrated by the process map from the organization's own website.

Division of Medical Quality Assurance Enforcement Process

It is as if the State is encouraging victims to simply give up. The title of this chart might as well be "Quit Now." Proceed with a complaint, however, and complainants will wait months for an anonymous probable cause panel to determine whether a complaint will be advanced for further review. Few complaints ever make it this far, and those that do rarely result in the Board of Medicine revoking a doctor's medical license.

I know most states' governors will not consider a singular action of revoking one doctor's medical license either popular or politically expedient. But they could, and they should.

Organizations like ChildUSA and others advocating for policy reform will continue to do their part and affect change. In Florida, these efforts will continue through efforts by people like State Senator Linda Stewart to pass "Donna's Law," Senate Bill 170. In 2020 this bill was signed into law by Florida Governor Ron DeSantis passed and made effective July 1, 2020. It closes the loophole in Florida's statute of limitations for child sex abuse that previously protected child sex abusers like Dr. Zink and others. While it will not apply retroactively, as it has in other states, this law will ensure that future perpetrators of child sex abuse will face certain justice if ever prosecuted.

I believe we are reaching a moment in society where more and more people are becoming aware and finding the courage to stand in solidarity with survivors of childhood sexual abuse. Perhaps someday these collective efforts will result in legislation that makes childhood sexual abuse a federal crime with no statute of limitations. States' rights and politics aside, I believe these changes are something that most Americans would agree are good for the country and its children.

I am hopeful. Changemakers are going to make change. Indeed, it is the only thing that ever will.

34
Hear Them Loud

What is it like to tell someone your story of childhood sexual abuse? What is the best way for people to respond? Two questions I've been asked a few times in one way or another by several people since I started talking about being sexually abused by my doctor as a child under the guise of medical care.

At its most basic level, I liken the experience of telling the story of my own childhood sexual assault to that of seeing a ghost and then telling someone about it. Knowing I saw something that was other-worldly, remembering the fear, questioning my own memory, and doubting whether anyone else would believe me. But I know what I saw, with my own eyes. And I know what I felt, on the back of my neck and in the pit of my stomach. It was real, but I can't prove it. No photo, no video, no audio recording. Just a memory, unmoored from the safe harbor it has taken for so many years. Ready to head back out to sea.

One idea I have meditated on is that the experience of telling someone about a story of childhood sexual abuse should be like introducing someone to an old friend. Meet my old friend. Yes, he is a grown man, with years of wisdom under his belt, with achievements and failures, with pride and regret. Meet my old friend, a soulful surfer who I knew best as a 16-year-old boy. He was the captain of my high school baseball team. A hard-working catcher who ran the game from behind the plate. He has a story to tell.

I have no reason NOT to believe him, so I will start by believing him and letting him know that I am here for him. I will listen to him tell me one of the most intimate and tragic stories he will ever tell, and I will tell him that it is not his fault. I will tell him that I am proud of him for trusting me with this information and for speaking his truth. I will ask him what I can do to help. Whatever he must tell me, I will not ask "Why?" Instead, I will hear him loud.

In the Fall of 2019, Stephanie and I traveled back to our beloved

Bakersfield, California to join friends for a concert at the Crystal Palace organized by Passing Through Productions and Guitar Masters. The Milk Carton Kids was the first band I pitched with the idea of playing Bakersfield as they were "passing through" on their 2013 tour. They took a pass then, but persistence paid off and they finally came around. It was a show for the ages.

In "Hear Them Loud" one of my favorite tracks off of their album The Ash & Clay, singers and guitarists Kenneth Pattengale and Joey Ryan deliver the following as a third verse followed by the chorus. It is a perfect answer for how to respond when someone tells you a story like mine.

> *My old friends they are few*
> *I still know them, they know me too*
> *Can't hear my tires hum in tune*
> *Far from home, I hope they're proud*
> *The ones you love*
> *Where are they now?*
> *The ones you love*
> *Where are they now?*
> *And I'm hoping that I'll still hear them loud.*

I hear you, old friend. I hope others do, too.

35

Epilogue: Words to My 16-Year-Old Self

My "Me Too" story began more than 30 years ago with a 16-year-old boy, crouched behind home plate – a crack of the bat, a violent play at the plate, and a world that would change forever. As I have shared my story, it has given me the opportunity to reflect on the characteristics of that 16-year-old boy that helped him to survive and thrive despite the awful trauma he experienced by being sexually abused and molested by someone he trusted. *Ambitious. Courageous. Focused. Humble. Integrity. Leader. Perseverant. Tenacious. Winner.* I can picture him in my mind, approaching the plate with his bat, his walk-up song "5 out of 6" by the Minneapolis rapper Dessa echoing through the stadium.

I'm the Phoenix, and the ash.
Red eyes shining in the camera flash.
My secret is I don't keep none,
See something go ahead and say something
I ain't afraid of it.
I don't drown, won't stay down
Heat finds a way to rise somehow.
Scan the crowd as I'm coming out and I
Don't see too many rivals now.

This kid is destined for greatness. Nothing can stop him. He will survive and thrive.

When I began sharing my story publicly through a daily blog post in February of 2020, I knew that it would be important to stay in the moment of each day and be mindful of how my story was received by others and how their responses affected me. Perhaps it would help me to become more empathetic, or at the very least, offer a perspective on how victims of childhood sexual assault and molestation might be supported. The following is a stream-of-consciousness list of notes I kept

130

on my phone during the weeks that followed the day I shared my story publicly. The note is titled "What Has Helped."

Stephanie's love and support. Colin and Olivia's love, support and "acting normal." A bike ride with Grant. Kindness of my co-workers. My therapist's encouragement. Facebook comments from friends expressing belief, love, and support. Emails and texts from Hawaii, Alaska, Oregon, California, Montana, Texas, Chicago, New Orleans, the Mississippi Delta, New England, NYC, New Jersey, Washington D.C., North Carolina, Florida, London. A fierce response from middle school friends. Rest. A brother's love. A shared reflection by Yung Pueblo that "A hero is one who heals their own wounds and then shows others how to do the same." Surfing buddies. Empathetic ears over the airwaves. Breakfast with Dad. That line from A Farewell to Arms, "The world breaks everyone, and afterward, some are strong at the broken places." The ocean and the waves.

My takeaway from these notes is the perspective that help did not come from some grand intervention or a final act of justice. It came in the form of everyday people doing everyday things, with empathy and kindness. It is a powerful lesson and a standard that I will try to bear for the rest of my life.

Throughout my adult life, whenever I have been faced with a challenge that appears insurmountable, I have turned to Galway Kinnell's poem "Another Night in the Ruins," for courage and inspiration. I am particularly moved by the seventh stanza that reads:

How many nights must it take
one such as me to learn
that we aren't, after all, made
from that bird that flies out of the ashes,
that for us
as we go up in flames, our one work
is
to open ourselves, to be
the flames?

These words are not a salve to allay my fears, but a stark reminder that the only way for me to live my life in service of the things that matter to me is to go "all in." To feel the deep pain of the trauma I have experienced and, while not wanting to live it again, to know that I am better at the broken places.

Sharing my story to help others and hopefully affect change someday has required everything of me and then some. Now that you know, it will inevitably require the same of you.

36

Resources

I f you are like me, an adult male survivor of childhood sexual abuse, one of the most important decisions I made was to talk to someone I could trust about my experience. In my case, I talked to my wife first, and eventually to a trained counselor and my primary care physician. The following are four resources that I found helpful that provide assistance to survivors of sexual abuse.

RAINN's National Sexual Assault Hotline

Whether you are looking for support, information, advice or a referral, RAINN's trained support specialists can help online at *www.rainn.org* or by calling 1.800.656.HOPE(4673).

1in6.org

If you are a man who has experienced sexual abuse or assault, you are not alone. At least 1 in 6 have experienced the same. *1in6.org* is here to support you in your path to a happier, healthier future.

CHILD USA

CHILD USA is the leading national think tank fighting for the civil rights of children. The organization's mission is to employ in-depth legal analysis and cutting-edge social science research to protect children, prevent future abuse and neglect, and bring justice to survivors. More information about its work, including child sex abuse statute of limitations reform can be found at *www.childusa.org*.

EMDR

EMDR (Eye Movement Desensitization and Reprocessing) is a psychotherapy that enables people to heal from the symptoms and emotional distress that are the result of disturbing life experiences. Repeated studies show that by using EMDR therapy people can experience the benefits of psychotherapy that once took years to make a difference. It is widely assumed that severe emotional pain requires a long time to heal. EMDR therapy shows that the mind can in fact heal from psychological trauma much as the body recovers from physical trauma. When you cut your hand, your body works to close the wound. If a foreign object or repeated injury irritates the wound, it festers and causes pain. Once the block is removed, healing resumes. EMDR therapy demonstrates that a similar sequence of events occurs with mental processes. The brain's information processing system naturally moves toward mental health. If the system is blocked or imbalanced by the impact of a disturbing event, the emotional wound festers and can cause intense suffering. Once the block is removed, healing resumes. Using the detailed protocols and procedures learned in EMDR therapy training sessions, clinicians help clients activate their natural healing processes.

More than 30 positive controlled outcome studies have been done on EMDR therapy. Some of the studies show that 84%-90% of single-trauma victims no longer have post-traumatic stress disorder after only three 90-minute sessions. Another study, funded by the HMO Kaiser Permanente, found that 100% of the single-trauma victims and 77% of multiple trauma victims no longer were diagnosed with PTSD after only six 50-minute sessions. In another study, 77% of combat veterans were free of PTSD in 12 sessions. There has been so much research on EMDR therapy that it is now recognized as an effective form of treatment for trauma and other disturbing experiences by organizations such as the American Psychiatric Association, the World Health Organization and the Department of Defense. Given the worldwide recognition as an effective treatment of trauma, you can easily see how EMDR therapy would be effective in treating the "everyday" memories that are the reason people have low self-esteem, feelings of powerlessness, and all the myriad problems that bring them in for therapy. Over 100,000 clinicians throughout the world use the therapy. Millions of people have been treated successfully over the past 25 years.

EMDR therapy is an eight-phase treatment. Eye movements (or other bilateral stimulation) are used during one part of the session. After the clinician has determined which memory to target first, he asks the client to hold different aspects of that event or thought in mind and to use his eyes to track the therapist's hand as it moves back and forth across the client's field of vision. As this happens, for reasons believed by a Harvard researcher to be connected with the biological mechanisms involved in Rapid Eye Movement (REM) sleep, internal associations arise, and the clients begin to process the memory and disturbing feelings. In successful EMDR therapy, the meaning of painful events is transformed on an emotional level.

For instance, a rape victim shifts from feeling horror and self-disgust to holding the firm belief that, "I survived it and I am strong." Unlike talk therapy, the insights clients gain in EMDR therapy result not so much from clinician interpretation, but from the client's own accelerated intellectual and emotional processes. The net effect is that clients conclude EMDR therapy feeling empowered by the very experiences that once debased them. Their wounds have not just closed, they have transformed. As a natural outcome of the EMDR therapeutic process, the clients' thoughts, feelings, and behavior are all robust indicators of emotional health and resolution—all without speaking in detail or doing homework used in other therapies.

More information can be found at *www.emdr.com.*

Green Shoe Foundation

The Green Shoe Foundation is a mental health non-profit organization offering adults over the age of 21 confidential, professional, five-day retreats aimed towards improving and impacting individual lives and communities. The goal of these retreats is to help participants embrace and heal the past, restore healthy patterns in life, create space to be your authentic self, and discover joy. Participants are empowered to experience personal growth, self-actualization, personal and professional success in forming and maintaining healthy relationships.

Green Shoe's five-day retreat is based on Post Induction Therapy, which originated from the experimental application of strategies developed to treat the effects of childhood relational trauma. These strategies were developed by Pia Mellody through her work at The Meadows inpatient treatment center.

Participation in Green Shoe's retreat is essentially free, primarily due to the generosity of Oklahoma philanthropist Chad Richison. A $475 deposit is refunded upon completion of the retreat by each participant.

More information can be found at *www.greenshoe.org.*

www.ingramcontent.com/pod-product-compliance
Lightning Source LLC
Chambersburg PA
CBHW020815300326
41914CB00081B/2009/J